GOLD

The Olympic Journey
of Daniel Ståhl & Vésteinn Hafsteinsson

by Vésteinn Hafsteinsson
with Dan McQuaid

This book is dedicated to Shaun Pickering,
a big man with a bigger heart.

PREFACE

by Dan McQuaid

The first international athletics championships I attended in person were the 2014 Europeans in Zurich. My wife's brother lives in the nearby town of Winterthur—I married wisely—and I was able to use his flat as a home base while commuting to Letzigrund Stadium to watch some of the world's best throwers ply their trade. At the time, I was most excited to see Robert Harting, the defending World, Olympic, and European champion, go up against Gerd Kanter and Piotr Malachowski in a battle of discus titans. Since the 2007 Worlds, competitions featuring those gents had been fiercely contested and fiercely entertaining. As a bonus, they typically ended with Robert ripping off his shirt and careening around the arena barbarian-style.

Robert did end up taking gold at those Euros, but unusually cold, damp conditions kept the distances fairly low—his winning mark was 66.07m—and I went home a little disappointed at having witnessed the least dramatic of his many triumphs.

It would be years before I realized that I'd actually seen something quite special at the 2014 Euros. Group A of the men's discus qualification marked the major championships debut of the world's next great discus thrower—the young Swedish giant, Daniel Ståhl.

I was aware at the time that Daniel had made a huge breakthrough earlier in the season with a throw of 66.89m. I was also aware that he was coached by Vésteinn Hafsteinsson, the man who guided Gerd Kanter to Olympic and World Championship gold. But that day in Zurich, Daniel stood out mainly for his size. Elite men's discus throwers tend to be large but lean. Imagine a high jumper after a couple years of protein shakes and power lifting. But Daniel looked mountainous, as if he'd wandered in from a local strongman competition. He also seemed tentative, and his performance that day—a best of 59.01m—made me wonder if the 66.89m had been a one-off product of the California winds.

By the time I attended another European Championships four years later in Berlin where my wife's sister has an apartment—Did I mention that I married wisely?—I knew how wrong I'd been in dismissing Daniel's potential. Since I'd seen him in Zurich, Daniel had developed into one of the world's top throwers, and he came into the 2018 Europeans as a World Championships silver medalist with a PB of 71.29m.

By then, the era of Harting and Kanter had passed, leaving Daniel and Lithuania's Andrius Gudžius as the new Übermenschen of the event. They had gone toe-to-toe at the 2017 Worlds, with Gudžius taking the gold by a mere two centimeters, and they put on another compelling show in Berlin with Gudžius once again finishing on top, in this case with a best throw of 68.46m to Daniel's 68.23m.

I spoke to Daniel afterwards in a chaotic and sweltering mixed zone. Berlin was in the middle of an historic heatwave, and the contest with Gudžius must have been exhausting, but Daniel exuded fierce energy as he leaned to speak into my microphone. "I'm very happy," he declared. "My goal was to win, but I'm proud of 68.23m. Now, I prepare to win in Doha!"

That was a reference to the upcoming 2019 World Championships where Daniel would, in fact, take the gold medal after putting together one of the greatest seasons in discus history.

In just five years, Daniel had grown from overmatched rookie to unstoppable discus force, and he was now the prohibitive favorite to take gold at the 2020 Olympics. But then...

When the pandemic hit in March of 2020, my friend Roger Einbecker and I reached out to coaches all over the world and asked them to participate in live webinars on the throwing events—a little something to lighten those dark days for coaches and throws enthusiasts isolating at home and missing the sport.

Several prominent names agreed to appear, including Mike Barber, Klaus Bartonietz, Uwe Hohn, Scott Bennett, Lance Deal, René Sack, and Vésteinn Hafsteinsson.

I was excited to get Vésteinn, but also nervous. I knew he was a native of Iceland, where it's always cold except when the volcanoes erupt, and there's something about those harsh, Nordic winters that seems to make people tightlipped and dour. Can you name a comedian from Iceland? Norway? Finland? Me neither.

I was worried when I called Vésteinn for a pre-webinar interview that I might not be able to get him talking. Luckily, I had a secret weapon at my disposal—my wife, Alice, who happens to be the world's friendliest person. Having a chat with Alice is like finding a twenty-dollar bill on the ground. No matter how grouchy you were previously, you walk away feeling good. Not even her tendency, as a lawyer of wills and trusts, to insert the topic of death randomly into conversations can spoil the effects of her charm.

And, funny thing, during the 1980's Alice briefly attended the University of Alabama, which just happens to be the alma mater of...Vésteinn Hafsteinsson.

Long story short, when I called Vésteinn to plan the webinar, I handed the phone off straight away to Alice. She got him laughing and sharing memories of Tuscaloosa, and we all had a lovely conversation.

A couple of weeks later, several hundred people from around the world joined Roger, Vésteinn, and me for an entertaining Zoom presentation on Daniel's technique. Afterwards, Roger and I thanked Vésteinn, congratulated ourselves on a big success, and went on with our lives.

But that fall, as the pandemic continued, we met with Vésteinn and two of his dear friends and collaborators, Hans Üürike and Shaun Pickering, to discuss the possibility of working on a long-delayed project of theirs: a comprehensive book covering Vésteinn's career as an athlete and coach.

It's not often that the most successful throws coach in the world asks you to write a book with him, so after thinking it over for approximately two seconds, Roger and I agreed.

In December, we began regular Zoom meetings—Vésteinn from Växjö, Sweden, Roger and I from our homes in the suburbs of Chicago—during which Vésteinn told us the story of his life, his career, and his philosophy of training. Over those cold, weird winter months as 2020 turned into 2021, Vésteinn spoke of his childhood in the small town of Selfoss where they had one TV channel, one radio channel, and every sport imaginable.

He told us about life in his big family. As was common in those days, his mother, Ragnhildur Ingvarsdóttir, managed the house, cooking every meal and somehow finding time to make clothes for Vésteinn and his four siblings. Meanwhile, Vésteinn's father devoted himself to making life in Selfoss richer for everyone. Besides working as a hospital administrator, Hafsteinn Þorvaldsson (Thorvaldsson) helped run local and regional sports clubs, held political office, and wrote for the local newspaper. The 2,500 residents of Selfoss were not enough to attract professional entertainers, so they had to put on their own shows to help pass the long winter nights, and Hafsteinn Þorvaldsson led the way. He taught himself how to dance and to play half a dozen musical instruments, taught others to dance and play those instruments and wrote encouraging reviews of local amateur theater performances, which he always described as "unbelievably good." Hafsteinn Þorvaldsson was, in Vésteinn's words, a "positive reinforcer."

Vésteinn spoke of his beloved older brother, Þráinn (Thrainn), an outstanding decathlete who taught him everything about sports. It was only natural for Vésteinn to follow his big brother to the University of Alabama, and it was there, at a party, that he met Anna Östenberg, a Swedish discus thrower who had just arrived on campus. Her first impression of Vésteinn? "Very big, and very blonde." They have been together ever since.

He described his long career as a thrower during which he represented Iceland at four Olympics and five World Championships, and he reminisced about his struggles to make a living as a coach while also managing the responsibilities of a husband and father. Maintaining a balance between family and career was, he said, the hardest challenge he faced.

The specter of Covid still loomed as we continued Zooming through the winter of 2021, and we spoke often of the upcoming season and the prospects for Vésteinn's group of throwers. Would the Olympics go on as scheduled? Could Daniel maintain his edge and take the gold medal in Tokyo? Might Simon Pettersson finish in the top five and set himself up to contend in 2024? And what of Vésteinn's up-and-coming shot putters Fanny Roos and Marcus Thomsen?

It was fascinating to have an inside look at how Vésteinn managed the challenges of that season which, as we now know, could hardly have turned out better. Fanny threw well in Tokyo and finished 7th. Daniel won discus gold. Simon, shockingly, took the silver medal.

Roger and I enjoyed a memorable Zoom with Vésteinn the day after the men's discus final. He was in his dormitory room in Tokyo, looking happy and exhausted and amazed as we congratulated him on his good fortune.

That was a giddy time for all of us, and for the world at large as vaccines and summer weather combined to make the pandemic seem a thing of the past.

But moving on turned out to be not so simple.

That fall, our meetings continued as Vésteinn went back to coaching his group in Växjö. But at some point, Roger began joining our calls from Arizona where he had gone to take care of his mother for what turned out to be the final weeks of her life. Shortly thereafter, he sold the insurance business he'd managed for many years and retired.

For a while, I still logged onto our meetings from my classroom at the high school where I'd taught English for nearly thirty years. But, exhausted by the pandemic and afraid that teaching would never be the same, I took a medical leave in January of 2022 and retired a few months later.

Vésteinn soldiered on with his group, but Fanny, Daniel, and Simon all struggled to find their form and it seemed like navigating the uncertainty of the previous two years while fighting their way to the top of the mountain might have left them drained.

We continued our Zooms throughout the 2022 season, and Vésteinn often appeared exhausted as well. Finally, on the day he was meant to fly to Eugene, Oregon, for the World Championships, he announced he would not be going. He remained home while his throwers traveled to America, and during that time had some serious discussions with Anna about his future in the sport.

Then, as the 2022 season ended, the Icelandic Sport and Olympic Association announced they were creating the position of Head of Elite Sports. Vésteinn had long dreamed of settling in Iceland after retiring from coaching and Anna, even though she was a native Swede, shared that desire. He asked her if he should apply.

"Yes," Anna told him. "Why not? Just for fun."

"I don't think I'll get it," he cautioned.

But a few weeks later, Vésteinn received a call from Iceland asking if he was serious about considering the position.

"I'm not sure," he replied. "Give me three days to think about it."

He decided to go ahead and interview, and by January of 2023 was in serious negotiations with the Icelandic Association. If Vésteinn agreed to a five-year contract, the job would be his.

As Head of Elite Sports, he would have a chance to exert a huge impact on the athletic culture in Iceland. He would be paid to help and encourage people the way his father had. He would be freed from the constant travel that had characterized his three decades as a coach. And, most importantly, he would make Anna happy. She had supported Vésteinn through many difficult days during his career but felt in her heart that another year on the road might literally kill him.

And so, at the top of his game, Vésteinn decided to step away from coaching. By the time you read this, he will have begun his new job in Iceland, and Daniel, Simon, Fanny, and Marcus will have moved on to other training groups, other mentors.

Roger, Vésteinn, and I still Zoom regularly and hope to produce more books. We decided that telling Daniel's story—which we believe many will find inspiring—was a great place to start, but it is just one episode from Vésteinn's career, and there are other adventures we plan to recount as well.

As for my original worries that Vésteinn might be one of those grim Nordic types, it turned out I was wrong. He for sure has a streak of Viking toughness running through him. But he's also kind and funny, principled and sentimental, and if there is one good thing that came to Roger and to me from the grim tumult of these last few years, it is that we can now call him our friend.

Acknowledgements

We owe thanks to many.

Hans Üürike and the late Shaun Pickering for providing the impetus to get this project moving.

The friends and colleagues of Daniel Ståhl who shared their memories with us.

Mike McQuaid for his design work.

The Estonian statistician Priit Tänava, who provided the statistics found at the back of this book, and who has made a huge contribution to the sport of discus throwing.

Arwid Koskinen for sharing many excellent photos.

Roger Einbecker who, besides taking on all of the technical aspects of turning a lot of stories, numbers and pictures into a book, was a calm and reassuring presence during this whole crazy process, though he could never quite keep his dogs quiet during Zooms.

And our wives, Anna Hafsteinsson Östenberg, Alice Wood, and Nancy Einbecker for their support and encouragement, and for pretending not to miss us during the hours we spent sequestered in Zoomland.

And to Daniel Ståhl himself, for letting us tell his remarkable story.

Introduction

by Vésteinn Hafsteinsson

When I first met Daniel Ståhl in 2009, he was a talented kid with an uncertain future. Partly, this was because of his size. He loved to throw the discus, but the top discus guys in those days—Gerd Kanter, Robert Harting, Virgilijus Alekna and Piotr Malachowski—were between 1.95m-2.03m (6'4"-6'8") tall and weighed around 130 kilos (286 lbs.). Daniel, at nineteen years old, already outweighed them by 30 kilograms! He moved well in the ring, but most coaches considered him too big to ever be a great discus thrower and thought he had more potential as a glide shot putter. They also questioned his work ethic. Daniel loved to laugh and have fun, and at times he did not seem to take his training seriously.

Later, I will tell the story of how I ended up meeting Daniel and becoming his coach. It was similar to my first meeting with Gerd Kanter in 2000. Nobody in Estonia wanted to coach Gerd, but I ended up taking him on after Raul Rebane, the Estonian sports journalist, convinced me to travel to Tallinn for a meeting. I saw something in Gerd that day, an immense passion that told me he could be special. Eight years later, he won Olympic gold.

The day I met Daniel, I saw that he burned with the same kind of fire. Daniel was a little younger than Gerd was when I met him, and a little less mature, but to me his potential was obvious. We just had to find a way to channel his energy into the discus.

It turned out that my journey with Daniel would be more successful and much more difficult than I imagined on the day I first traveled to Stockholm to watch him train. Over the next decade, he would become one of the greatest discus throwers in history, a World and Olympic champion like Gerd, and a hero to many people in Sweden and in Finland--his mother's home country. But in order to reach that level, Daniel had to endure years of disappointment and self-doubt.

I hope this story will inspire those embarking on their own journey whether in athletics or other fields. Daniel's courage and persistence as he fought through many dark days are something we all can strive to emulate.

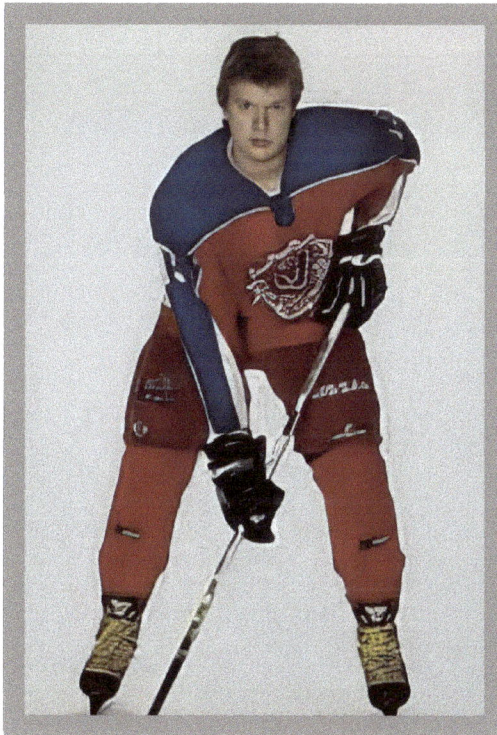

The young hockey player Ståhl that decided to be a discus thrower

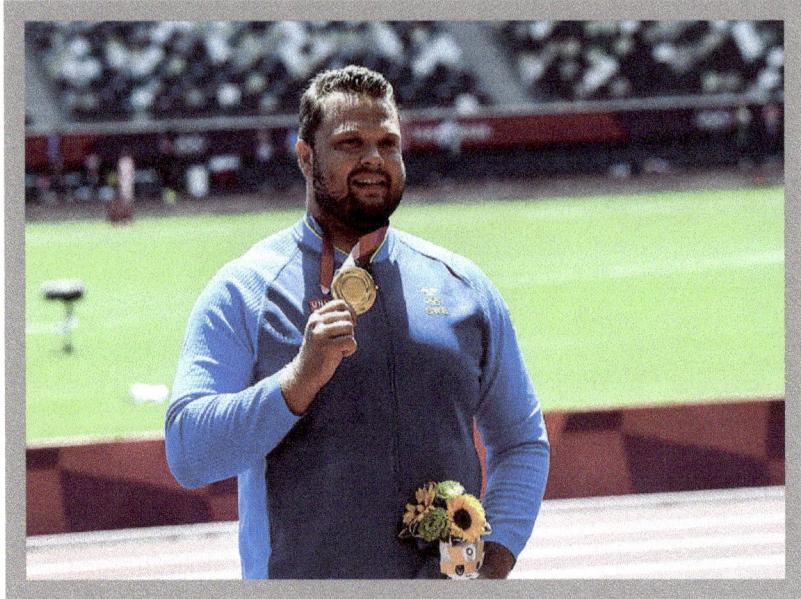

Daniel Ståhl, the 2020 Olympic Gold Medalist

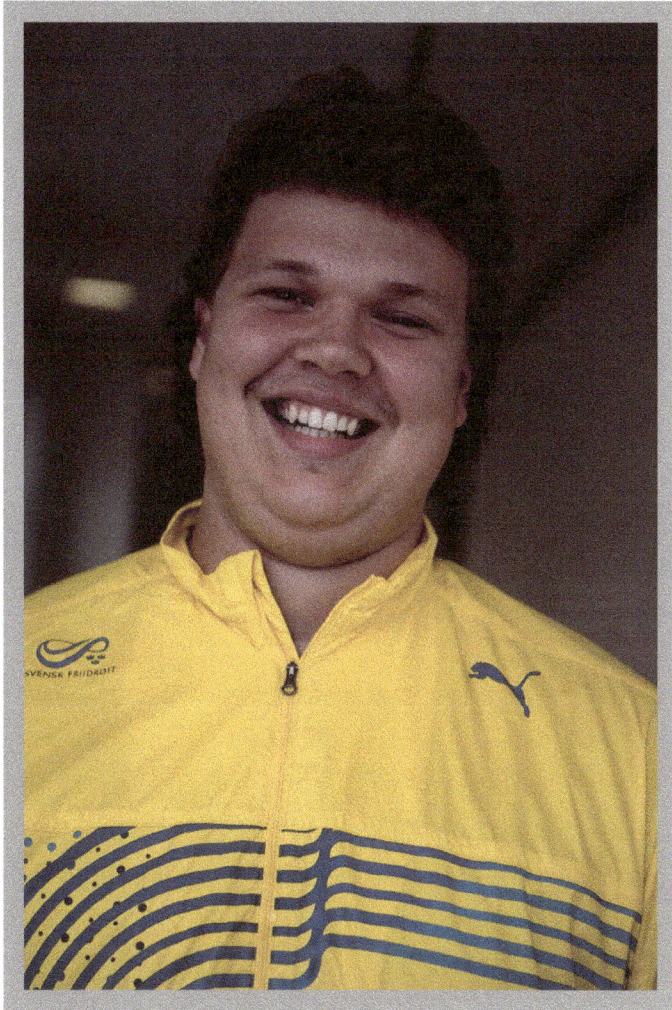

Daniel Ståhl, ready to begin his discus journey.

1

And So It Begins

Here is the story of how I became the coach of Daniel Ståhl.

In 2009, I was living in Växjö, Sweden, and working with a group of athletes from all over the world including Gerd Kanter, the defending Olympic champion in the discus. Nik Arrhenius was also in that group, and he and his younger brother Leif started telling me about a big kid from their athletics club, Spårvägen in Stockholm, who had potential as a discus thrower. The kid's name was Daniel Ståhl.

The situation reminded me of when I first heard about Gerd in the fall of 2000. Out of the blue, a sports journalist named Raul Rebane called from Estonia to ask me to come meet some kid who was looking for a coach.

Raul had seen Gerd throw a couple of times, then one day ran into him on the street in Tallinn. They sat down to chat, and Gerd told Raul that all he wanted in life was to be a great athlete. As a kid, Gerd loved basketball and hoped to be the next Michael Jordan, but by the time he met Raul, he had transferred his passion to the discus. Only he was

Mac Wilkins
on developing Daniel's talent

" It's always interesting when you look at an athlete and try to project their potential and evaluate any shortcomings that might hold them back. Daniel already had some decent results when I met him, and the first thing you see with him is his physical size. And he had the strength, or was developing the strength, to be a world beater.

What you always wonder, though, is does the athlete have the persistence to fail enough to get better? That can be a tough one. You've got to be able to handle not doing it right and have the desire and persistence to ultimately *get* it right.

The next question is, what is his mental capacity for competing? That's something that can be developed over time, but it's not easy. It involves the athlete and the coach working endlessly to find the effortless throw.

It turned out that Vésteinn was the right person to guide Daniel through that process. They met, and the rest is history. "

twenty-one years old with no funding, no coach, and no training plan. He did not even own a decent discus or nice pair of throwing shoes because he could not afford them and was not considered promising enough to receive support from the Estonian federation. But for some reason, Gerd believed he would be a success, and Raul was inspired by Gerd's determination, so he decided to help him find a coach. Unfortunately, even though Raul was a very well-connected sports journalist and knew all the discus coaches in Estonia, he could not convince anyone to work with Gerd. They did not think a twenty-one-year-old with a PB of 53 meters had a future in the sport.

But Raul is a persistent guy, and he decided if he could not find Gerd a coach in Estonia, he would find one somewhere else. That summer, he spent a month in Sydney covering the Olympic Games, and while he was there, he talked to coaches from all over Europe—Finland, Germany, Sweden, Croatia—but nobody was interested. Then, one day he ended up sitting next to a broadcaster from Iceland, my native country. Raul asked the guy if he knew someone who might be willing to coach Gerd. "Well," the man replied, "I know only one discus coach, and that is Vésteinn Hafsteinsson."

Raul called me a couple of weeks later. "You don't know me," he said, "but I have a discus thrower for you—a young man with big hands!" I think he meant to say, "big wingspan," but regardless, Raul ended up convincing me to travel to Tallinn to meet Gerd.

When Raul told his wife I was coming, she was surprised. "He is traveling to Estonia because of a phone call from a person he never knew to see a person he doesn't know? This cannot be a normal man."

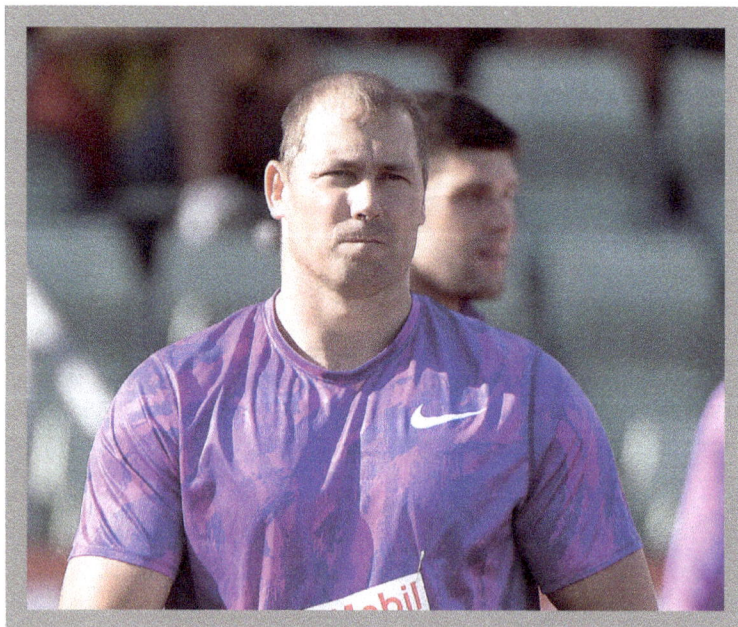

Gerd Kanter... my first World and Olympic champion. He and Daniel would have remarkably similar careers.

Looking back, I have to agree. I came to Tallinn in November of 2000 in the freezing cold, and Raul picked me up from the airport in his car. Estonia was still struggling then to recover from the years of Soviet domination, and everything seemed gray and worn down. It reminded me of East Germany when I competed there in the 1980's. Raul smoked the whole way to the training hall, which made me carsick. When we arrived at the facility, there was another car parked a few meters away. It was an old Lada, which also made me think of the Eastern Bloc. Next thing I knew, Gerd jumped out of the Lada and came walking towards me with his hand extended and his eyes popping out of his head. Looking very intense, he shook my hand and said, "Welcome to Tallinn, coach!

We went into the training hall, and I put Gerd through all kinds of tests. The results indicated there was nothing special about him physically, except for his speed in the sprints.

Niklas Arrhenius
on young Daniel

66 Daniel's parents and my parents were in the same track club. My dad was born and raised in Stockholm, and he joined the Spårvägen club when he was twenty-one and just out of the military. Daniel's dad was a hammer thrower for Spårvägen, and his mom threw for them as well. I grew up in the United States, but every summer we'd visit Sweden and when we did, we'd always have dinner at the Ståhl's house. Daniel's mom, Taina, was a Swedish-speaking Finn, and she made Finnish dishes that my dad loved. I remember when Daniel was around thirteen years old, he passed me in height—and I was a grown man who had already thrown the discus 60 meters! He was obsessed with hockey then, but I kept telling him, "Dude, you're a big guy and you're going to get bigger. Try throwing. That's your future." 99

He had a terrible feeling for the discus, an average overhead shot put throw, and low numbers in the jumps. But I immediately agreed to coach him because of the passion he showed that day. It's hard to explain, but the look in Gerd's eyes told me he had a chance to achieve something great.

In 2007, after years of work and many hard lessons, Gerd became World Champion. In 2008, he won Olympic gold.

Then, a decade after I met Gerd, the Arrhenius brothers thought they might have found another "diamond in the rough."

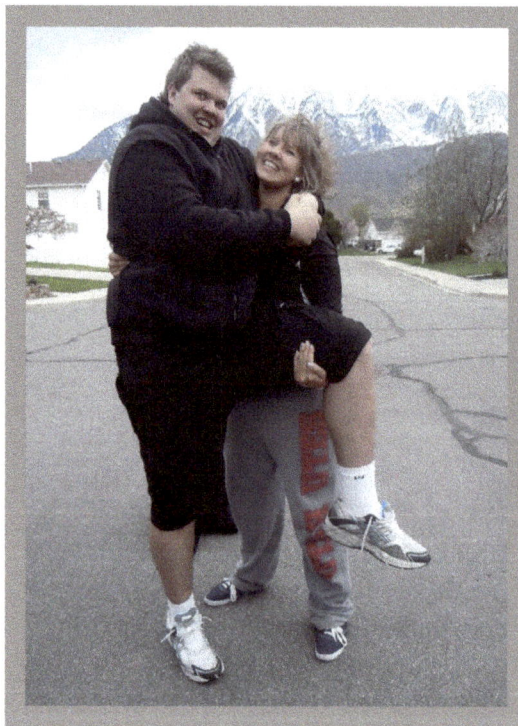

Daniel and his older sister, Anneli, who was a hammer thrower at University of Utah

So, one day in the fall of 2009, I stopped by the indoor facility where their club trained. Åke Ruus, the throwing coordinator at Spårvägen, arranged for me to come and watch Daniel throw. When I walked in, there was Daniel, a huge, out-of-shape kid dressed in a black Adidas uniform. He seemed shy and barely said a word when we were introduced. Then, he started to laugh for no apparent reason.

Arwid Koskinen
on competing against Daniel

66 The first time I saw Daniel was at a competition when we were young. I hated to lose, so when I arrived and saw this big guy, like 1.92m tall, I thought, "I hope he's in the senior division." Then, when I found out we were the same age, I almost started crying.

We competed against each other in the shot put while we were growing up, and we were usually pretty even, so we pushed each other to make better results. After a while, we began training with the same coach, the shot putter Hans Almström. I was better than Daniel in training because I was always pumped up to throw far in practice while Daniel was more focused on throwing far in competitions.

One year at youth nationals, he was right in front of me in the order, and each round he was throwing farther, and then I was throwing farther. He went ahead in the last round and was so happy that he came at me and jumped like I was supposed to catch him. He weighed around 140 or 150 kilos, and I was like, "Daniel! I can't catch you!"

Then, on my last attempt, I threw farther than him, so I jumped into his arms—but it was easy for him to catch me. 99

When he got into the cage, he started firing discs every which way— into the net on the right, into the net on the left, straight up—the whole time screaming and laughing as if this was this was the most fun he'd ever had.

I had never seen a thrower like him. Daniel was a huge guy, but he had smooth moves in the ring and an energy level that was off the charts. He also had a 2.20m wingspan, which did not hurt.

Daniel had a reputation for acting immature, but that didn't worry me. I figured he would outgrow the kid stuff. What I needed to know was whether he was willing to put in the years of work it would take to get to the top. In size and athleticism, he was superior to Gerd, but would he work as hard as Gerd to make the most of his potential?

I knew Daniel's mom, Taina, was Swedish discus champion in 1987, and his father, Jan, had competed in the hammer, so I thought there must be some toughness and discipline in Daniel's DNA.

Elias Håkansson
on his first impressions of Daniel

66 My first memories of Daniel involve the kind of awkward teenage moments that people cringe about until the day they die. One came in 2010 when Arwid, Daniel and I all made the team for the Junior Worlds in Moncton, Canada. While we were there, Daniel did laundry and put a shirt on a hanger which he hung on the head of the fire sprinkler in his room. At some point, he realized he was late for a training session, and as he rushed out of his room, he tried to pull the shirt off the hanger. But the shirt stuck to the hanger, and he ended up breaking open the sprinkler head. Every room on the entire floor got flooded. People had to wade through five inches of water in the hallway. The fire department came, and they evacuated the entire building. The place was a complete mess! But it was on the Moncton trip where Daniel and I got to know each other. Soon after, I joined his club, Spårvägen, and we've been friends ever since. 99

I ended up coming back and doing a session with Daniel whenever I was in Stockholm, maybe six sessions over the winter of 2010-2011. By the summer of 2011, I decided he and I needed to have a serious talk.

One day when I was in Stockholm watching Daniel throw, I asked Taina and Jan if I could have a private moment with their son. Daniel and I went for a little walk, and I put it to him straight.

"You are a fool," I told him.

"What do you mean?" he asked.

"You have the talent to be a great athlete, but you'd rather hang out with your friends and eat junk food and goof around all day. Now, do you want to spend your life wasting time, or do you want to be the best discus thrower in the world?"

Daniel was surprised to hear me talk this way, and at first, he just laughed.

But I didn't laugh, and after a moment he understood this was a turning point. If he wanted to take this journey with the idea of going all the way, then I would go with him. If not, it was time to end our collaboration. I would return to Växjö, and he could go on with his life in Stockholm.

After considering for a few moments, he spoke. "I want to be the best discus thrower in the world!"

"Good," I replied. "Then you must do what I say, and you must be ready to work hard for eight or ten years, because that is how long it will take."

This was a lot to swallow for a kid who up until then had probably never considered his future.

"Okay," he finally said. "I will do it."

And that is how I became the coach of Daniel Ståhl.

Shaun Pickering
on young Daniel

" Daniel was the only athlete Vésteinn ever recruited. His reputation was that he was a bit unruly and difficult to work with. Part of this might have been because he was so massive. Daniel loved playing hockey when he was growing up, and later, after he and Vésteinn had been together for a while, he presented Vésteinn with one of his old training shirts—it was a 9XL. Basically, Daniel was a fun character who liked to make people laugh, but when you're his size, it's easy for people to get intimidated. Vésteinn, though, was not intimidated. "

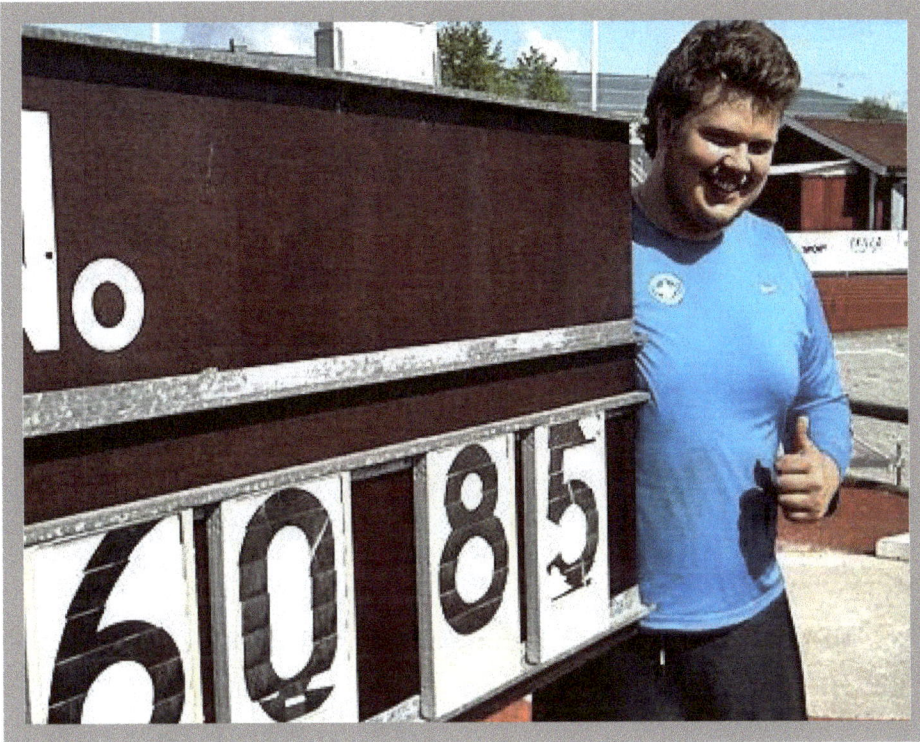

Daniel after throwing his personal best with the 1.75kg discus
as a Junior in 2011 in Bålsta, Sweden

2

2011 & 2012 —
Our First Year Together

My first task with Daniel was to get him into shape. When we began training together regularly in October of 2011, he was too heavy to handle all the reps we needed him to do in the discus ring. To remedy this, we started with a training program that consisted entirely of general preparation exercises: walking, medicine ball throws, gymnastics, circuit training, hurdle walks, and a little bit of throwing.

Daniel took a room in Växjö, and when we started, he would stay there a week or two each month, then go back to his parents' house in Stockholm. He called me from there after I sent him his first program.

"You want me to walk four times a week for an hour?"

"Yes."

"And no bench press for four weeks?"

"Correct."

"What kind of program is this?"

I had a similar conversation with his father.

"No bench press?"

"No."

"How will he throw farther if he loses strength?"

"You must believe me," I told him, "Your son will be very strong in the future, but I am the coach, and you are the father, and I will determine the program."

I had a similar situation with Gerd Kanter when I sent him his first program in 2000. Before he began training with me, Gerd mostly did bench presses and squats. This made his chest and rear end very big—Raul told him he looked like a pregnant duck—but it did not produce far throws, so we changed him to a more balanced program that included mobility and flexibility work. Instead of bench pressing four times a week as

Niklas Arrhenius
on Daniel's development

66 When he first started with Vésteinn, Daniel couldn't really do drills because he was so big and so undeveloped that his feet and ankles couldn't handle the load. He had to get stronger at the little places in his body, and he had a long way to go if he was ever going to succeed as a discus thrower. He was just a big, fun-loving kid, and nobody could tell for sure if he'd be able to change his diet and attitude and really go for it. Luckily, Vésteinn had the stubbornness and ability to get Daniel to commit. And once he did, Daniel started getting better right away. 99

he had been doing, I had Gerd bench press twice per week. This made him very unhappy. He became even less happy when I told him it might be years before he hit another bench press PB.

But I explained to Gerd that if he wanted to be a great discus thrower, we had to focus more on correcting his weaknesses such as his lack of flexibility and poor throwing technique and focus less on making him a champion bench presser. Besides, he could already bench 190 kilos, which was enough for him to throw far if he developed in other ways.

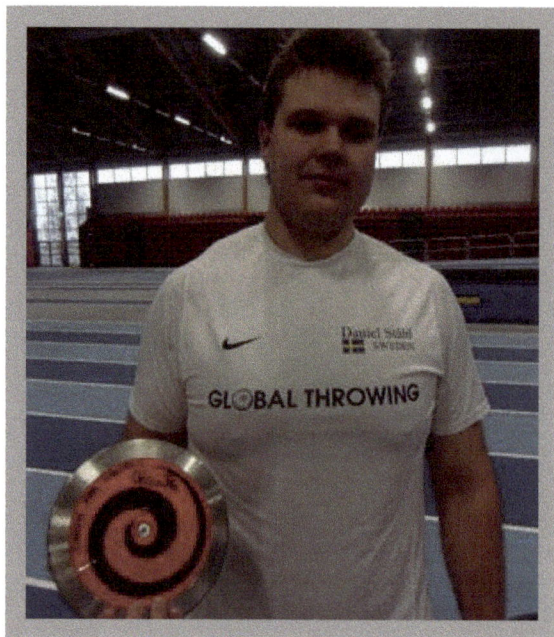

An autographed discus from Gerd Kanter

Once I explained this, Gerd trusted me and followed the programs I wrote for him faithfully for the next eight years—programs which always included 20-30 minutes of exercises to enhance his mobility and flexibility before every workout, something he'd have considered a waste of time before he started working with me.

It was the same way with Daniel.

"My goal for you," I told him, "Is to be the best discus thrower in the world someday. But first, you need to get fit. I am in charge now, and you have to trust me."

He accepted this, and we made a lot of progress that first year.

Another important part of getting Daniel into shape was changing his diet. He was a big guy with a big appetite who ate whatever he wanted and did not think about

> Vésteinn brought Daniel into the group and set about getting him into shape to train like a discus thrower. Daniel had great farmer's strength then, but he couldn't use it because he was so out of shape. He couldn't do the amount of throws he needed to do to learn technique. He couldn't even do many reps on throwing drills because his ankles couldn't take it, so Vésteinn had to tear him down to build him up.
>
> It was an interesting battle for a while because his mom and dad were from a powerlifting background—his mom was a powerlifting champion in Europe, and his dad was really strong, so they wanted Daniel to get bigger and stronger thinking it would make him throw farther. Vésteinn had to get Daniel's parents to accept the plan of "Let's get him athletic and teach him technique, and when he can handle sixty throws a day, then we'll get him stronger."

the consequences. The first thing I told him was he needed to start eating like a regular person. He would do his walking in the morning, then eat a normal-sized breakfast of only one portion. Lunch and dinner would consist of one third fish or meat, one third carbs like potatoes, rice, or pasta, and one third vegetables—again, one portion of each. Between meals, every three hours or so he could have some yogurt or fruit.

On special occasions, if he was invited to a birthday party or something, he could have some sweets, but not too many.

That first year, Daniel was very good at following these instructions. He called me once when he was about to go to a party where he knew there would be a lot of cakes.

"How am I going to do this?" he asked.

"Eat dinner first," I told him. "Then, at the party, eat just one piece of cake. Do not eat a whole cake."

It was not easy for Daniel to stick to a disciplined eating plan, but he did his best and lost 30 kilograms in eight months.

Not surprisingly, he lost some strength as well. In the spring of 2012, he struggled to complete three reps with 110 kilos in the bench press and could barely get through a set with 40 kilos in seated behind-the-neck press. For a guy his size, those were not impressive numbers, and it took a lot of faith for him to stick with the program.

Gerd Kanter
on young Daniel

I first started seeing Daniel at training camps and when Vésteinn would hold clinics in Sweden for juniors. I remember he was a big kid who was considered as a huge talent.

He was still just a kid when he joined the group in Växjö. One day, we were in a restaurant where they had a buffet and Daniel ate all the meatballs. The rest of us were a little mad at him because when you have a buffet there is always a certain calculation of how much you serve for a certain amount of people, and Daniel on his own took care of all the meatballs.

He was a little immature, but he was nineteen and I was thirty, so it is not too surprising that he would seem a little childish to me.

Generally, though, we had a very good kind of connection and always had a lot of fun. It was fun to make Daniel laugh, and after a while I started to feel like he was sort of a younger brother who was coming up. I could see that he had a bright future, and he for sure had the tools to someday be the best.

But he did stick with it, and by the time we traveled to California in April for a training camp, he was feeling fit and moving well. This allowed him to start throwing better, and he had a great summer of training. In August, he ended up finishing second at the Swedish Championships with a throw of 62.16m—a seven-meter increase from the previous year!

His father Jan was astonished. "I just don't get it," he said to me one day that summer. "How can he lose thirty kilograms and a bunch of strength and throw a seven-meter PB?"

But this was only the beginning. To keep improving, Daniel needed to develop socially also, and the first step was getting used to being away from his parents and all his friends in Stockholm.

Niklas Arrhenius
on Daniel's early struggles

66 When he first joined Vésteinn's group, I was the only person Daniel knew in Växjö. I think it was hard on him being away from home for the first time. He was young when he started training there, and he'd never really been away from home. I had gone to Sweden on a church mission for two years when I was his age, so I could relate a little bit to what he was feeling, and I just kept encouraging him. I became a voice in his head saying, "Hey man, you can handle the homesickness. You have this special potential. You can get to the top, and Vésteinn is the guy to take you there." I tried to be like a big brother to him. Sometimes, if Vésteinn was tough on him, I'd explain that it wasn't out of spite, it was because Vésteinn believed in him. I was ten years older than Daniel and had a lot more experience, and because we had known each other for so long, he trusted me. 99

This was difficult for him, probably harder than changing his diet. Daniel was always most comfortable when he was around his family and his Stockholm buddies, and he got very homesick whenever he stayed long in Växjö. I was worried at times that he might give up and move back home until Niklas Arrhenius came to train with us that summer.

As I mentioned, Daniel, Niklas, and Leif Arrhenius all competed for the Spårvägen club in Stockholm, and their families were old friends.

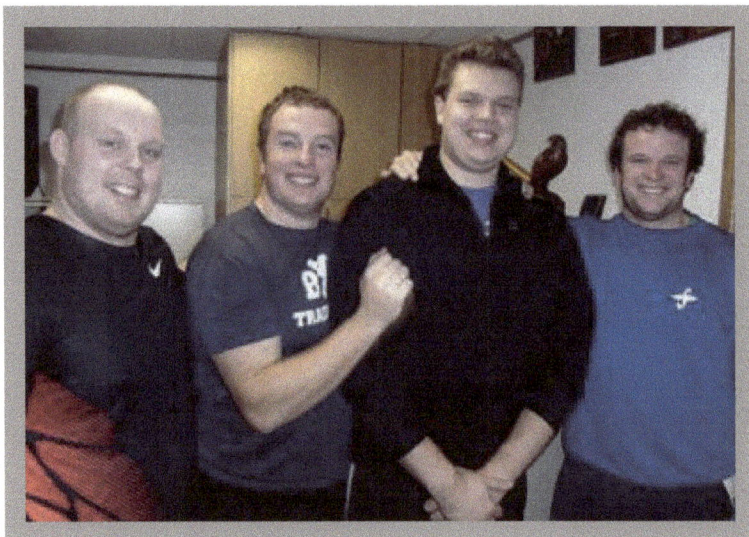

Kim Christensen, Nik Arrhenius, Daniel and Leif Arrhenius on a training camp in Provo, Utah, in January of 2012.

Daniel looked up to the Arrhenius brothers since he was a kid, so he was happy when Niklas came to Växjö and treated him almost like a son, encouraging him and giving him advice. Without the support he got from Niklas, I don't know if Daniel would have overcome his homesickness. His career might have ended before it began.

The payback for Niklas was that Daniel almost beat him at the Swedish Championships when he threw his 62.16m PB. Daniel was ahead most of the way until Niklas hit 62.32m in the final round to take the win.

All things considered, 2012 was a successful year for Daniel. He got in good shape and learned some things about life as a professional athlete. Overall, I was happy with his progress and with my decision to become his coach. I could tell, based on what I saw during our first year together, that Daniel had a chance to do great things.

Hans Üürike
on Daniel's showmanship

  I took over managing Daniel in 2012, and as part of his development I tried to get him to do smaller meets around Europe to get experience throwing in different conditions—rain, cold, big arenas, small arenas, whatever. He came to Estonia a few times, and in Tallinn he threw a 58.67m PB and then screamed like crazy and ran all over the stadium, still screaming. Everyone started looking and wondering what was going on in the discus for this guy to act this way, and that is when I first realized Daniel had the ability to make a whole stadium pay attention. This is a rare thing in the throws because they are hard for the average spectator to follow. Every idiot can understand who won a running event, but most spectators don't see the technical differences between a good and bad throw, so they get bored. With Daniel, though, the discus was never boring.

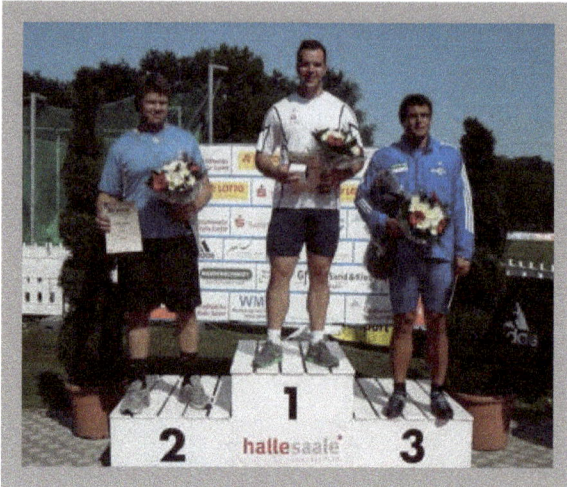

Daniel finished second
in this comp in Halle, Germany.
Lukas Weißhaidinger of
Austria won the competition
and Hendrik Müller of
Germany was third.

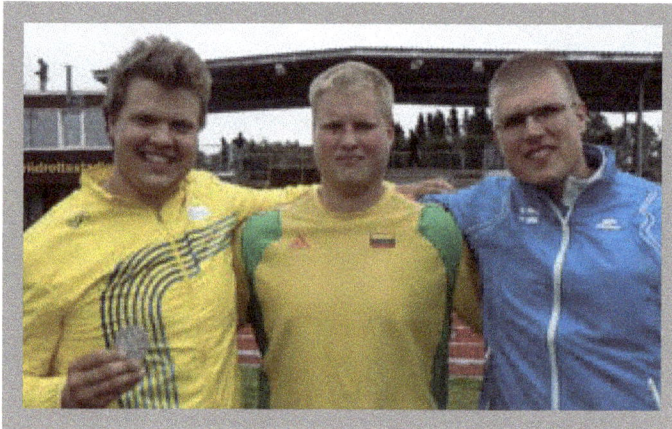

Daniel finished second
at a Nordic vs Baltic U22
meet in Jessheim,
Norway to Andrius Gudžius
of Lithuania (center).
Ville Kivioja of Finland
was third. Gudžius won
the meet, beating
Daniel 61.44 to 61.42

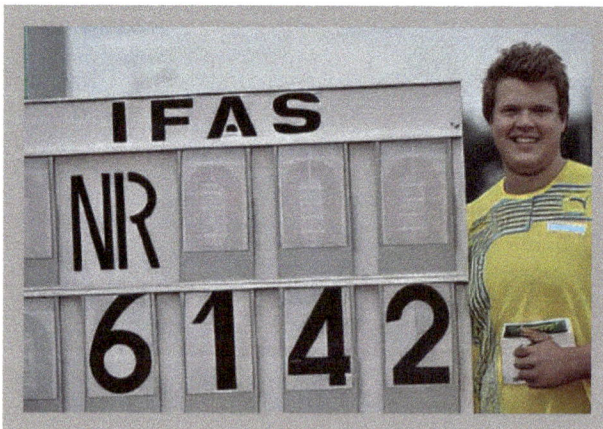

Daniel sets a
new personal best in
Jessheim in 2012

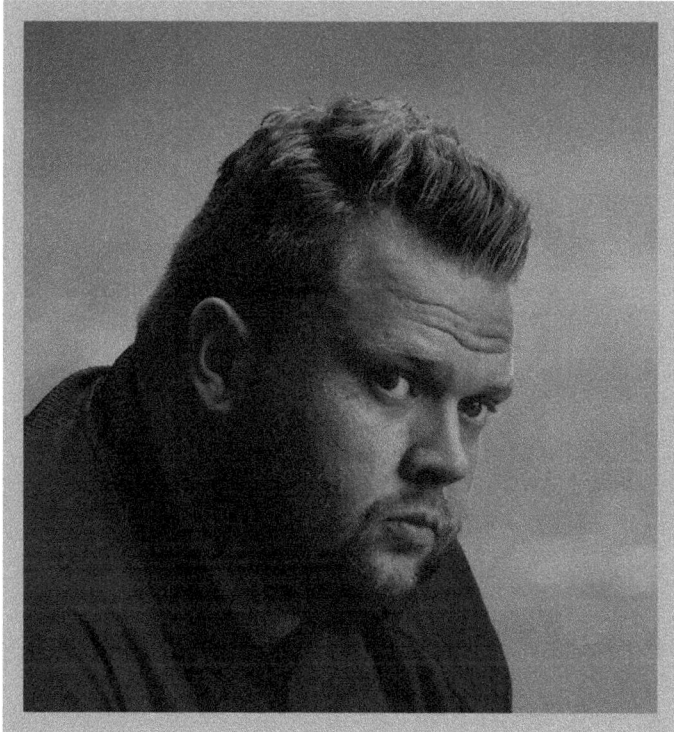

This is a picture of Daniel much later in his career when sometimes, in a quiet moment, we would sit back and reflect on all we'd been through.

3

2013 — A Year of Struggle

Coaching would be a lot easier if athletes always improved, getting a little bit better each year until they reached their peak. That's pretty much how things went with Gerd. Here are his season's best throws during the first six years we worked together:

2001: 60.47m
2002: 66.31m
2003: 67.13m
2004: 68.50m
2005: 70.10m
2006: 73.38m

Unfortunately, this doesn't happen for everyone, and after making a big jump in 2012, Daniel took a step back in 2013. His motivation wavered, and he never found his rhythm in the ring.

This surprised me. Daniel followed our plan faithfully during 2011-2012 and improved by nearly seven meters, so I expected him to be excited about taking the next step in 2013.

That's how it had been with Gerd. Once Gerd and I shook hands that day in Tallinn and started working together, his motivation never wavered. He wanted in every fiber of his body to be a great discus thrower, and he never doubted he was on the right path. His belief was confirmed by our early success, which made him want to work even harder and succeed more. When Gerd traveled to be with me for training, he would take a room nearby and after each session he would go back to his room and rest for the next session. He never got bored or restless, and he had no interest in doing anything other than training, resting, and dreaming about winning an Olympic gold medal.

That was Gerd's personality. He was serious, confident and extremely focused on his goal of becoming a great thrower.

But Daniel was different. He became bored very easily and did not like that there was very little to do in Växjö as compared to Stockholm.

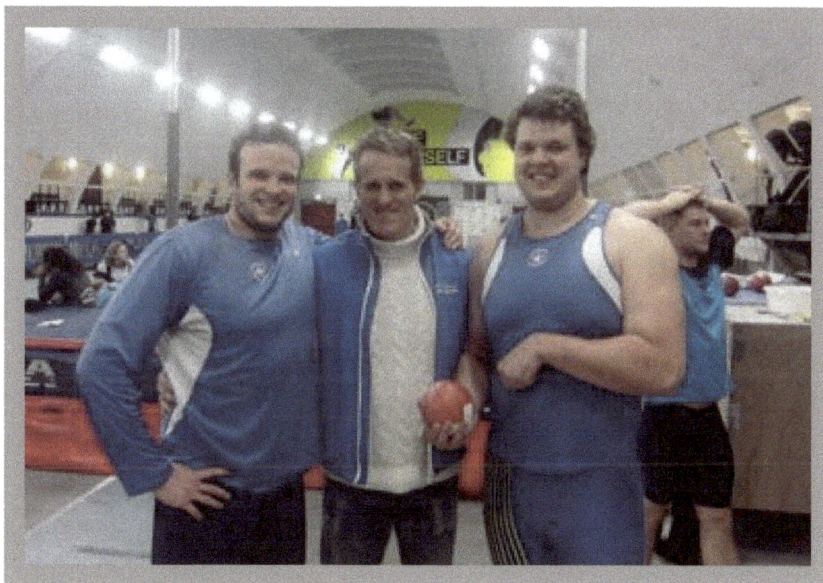

Photo courtesy of Vésteinn Hafsteinsson

Leif Arrhenius, Vésteinn and Daniel after a meet in the Sparta Hall in Copenhagen, Denmark

Nick Percy
on Daniel's development

" I first met Daniel in Halle in 2012, the year before I joined Vésteinn's group. Here was this huge, goofy, laughing guy throwing the disc, and I was like, "They make people this big?"

Then when I joined the group and started training with him, I saw how raw and undeveloped he was. When he threw, you never knew if the disc was going to end up in the ceiling or in the stands. But Vésteinn was the perfect coach for Daniel because he was relentless about teaching technique.

He used to coach me by Skype when I went to college at Nebraska. I'd set up my computer in the hallway of my freshman dorm and people would open their doors and see me spinning around and probably wonder, "Is this guy on crack?"

And there was Vésteinn's voice coming through the computer, "Do it again, Nick! The rhythm is one-two-three…" When the group was in Chula Vista, we'd drill next to a basketball court at the Foxwood apartments. Everyone struggled with the technique at first, but once in a while, you'd see a little flash of magic from Daniel and think, "Hmmmm." "

Daniel felt especially bored and lonely after Niklas Arrhenius returned to the United States in the fall of 2012. He began eating poorly again, and the weight he gained had a negative impact on his training. It also made him feel embarrassed. Gerd was no longer in our group, but Daniel had been around him enough over the previous two years to know how seriously Gerd took his job as a discus thrower. Now Daniel began to wonder whether he could ever be as disciplined as Gerd. He liked to have fun in whatever he did, but training, dieting and being away from home were not fun for him in 2013.

We went to California again that spring, but he did not have a good training camp, and he often felt down during the summer.

One positive development during the 2013 season came at the European Athletics U23 Championships, where Daniel threw a season's best of 61.29m to finish fourth against a field that included some guys who went on to be very successful like Andrius Gudžius, Viktor Butenko, Lukas Weißhaidinger and Philip Milanov.

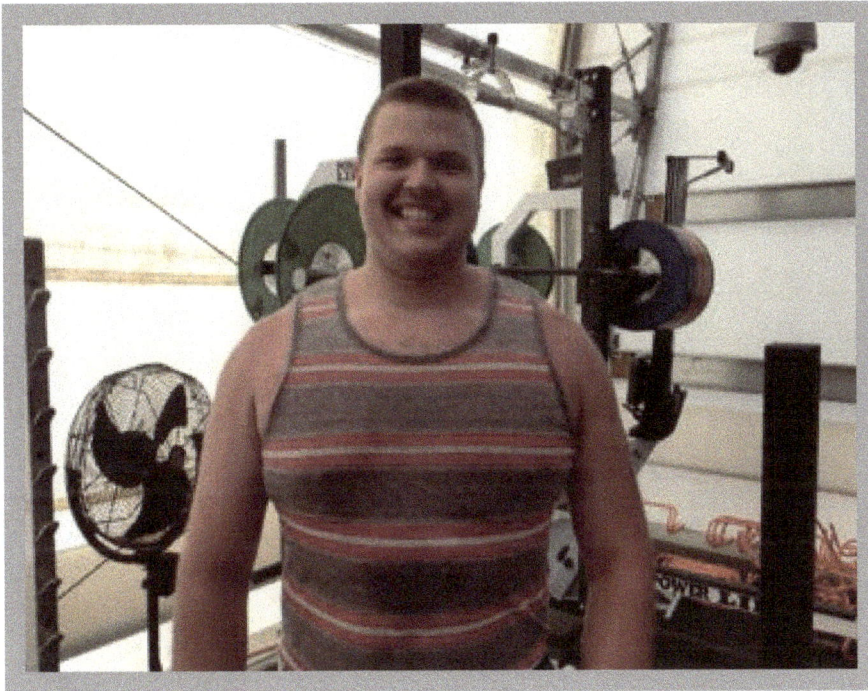

In the weight room in Chula Vista

This was Daniel's first success at an international championship at the junior level, and I hoped his performance there would lift his spirits and give him some momentum going into 2014.

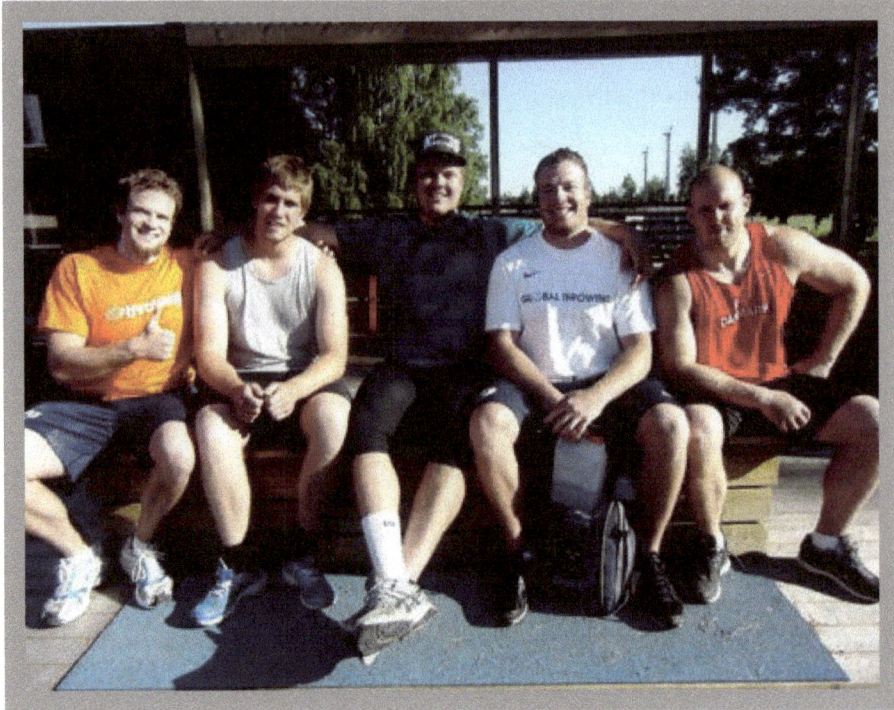

Leif Arrhenius, Viktor Gardenkrans, Daniel, Nik Arrhenius
and Kim Christensen at the throwing field in Växjö

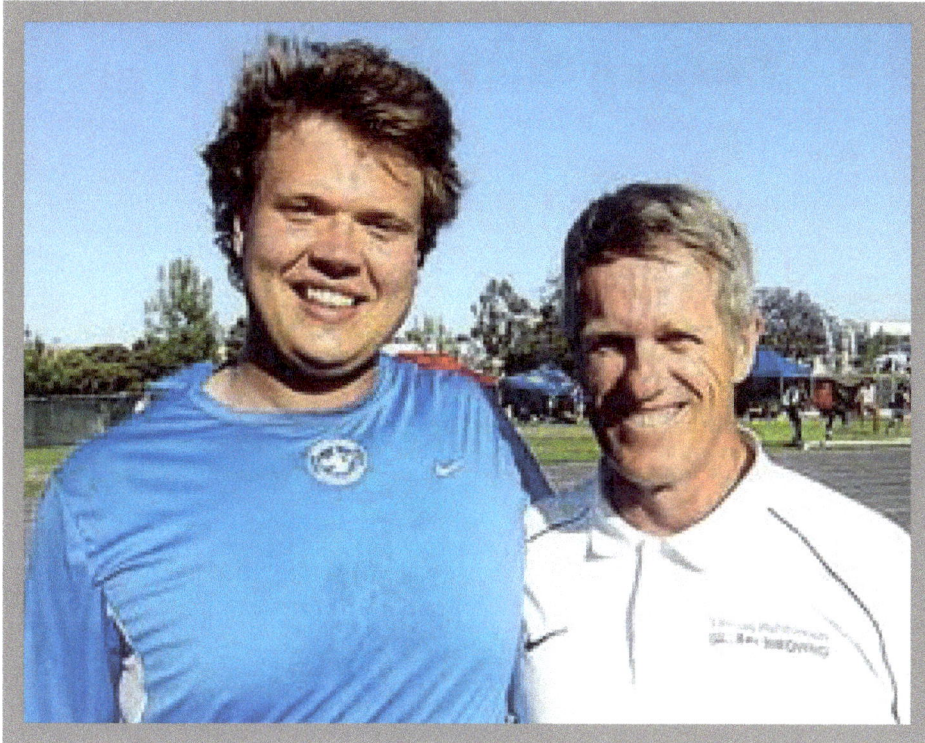

Daniel with a happy coach

## 4

2014 — A Huge Breakthrough and Painful Lesson

Daniel did seem to be more focused as we prepared for the 2014 season. He went back to eating a healthy diet, rediscovered his fitness and started moving very well again in the discus ring.

It was very helpful when the Swedish Olympic Committee put us together with a nutritionist named Linda Bakkman, who has worked with Daniel ever since. Linda taught Daniel how to eat like an athlete. She coached him on what to order at restaurants and what items to choose at a grocery store. When we traveled, Daniel started bringing snacks—bags of nuts and grapes or something—that he had prepared in advance for the trip. This was Linda's doing, and she made a big difference to Daniel over the course of his career.

In March of 2014, Daniel got second to Danijel Furtula in the U23 division at the European Winter Throwing Cup in Portugal. He only threw 57.70m, but this was his first medal at any kind of high-level international junior competition, so he was in good spirits when we traveled to California a couple of weeks later.

This time, training camp went well, and he threw a PB of 63.09m at a meet in Chula Vista. Then, on the third of May, we went to a competition in Irvine where the conditions were awful. The heat felt oppressive, especially for us who were used to the weather in Sweden. In order to stand it, we had to walk around with ice bags on our necks. There was no "California wind" that day, and I thought for a while maybe we should just pack it in and go home because for sure nobody would perform well.

Then Daniel threw 66.89m.

This throw is on Youtube, and if you watch it you can hear a crazy person screaming in the background. The crazy person was me.

Shaun Pickering
on the 66.89m throw

66 Daniel was in much better shape when Vésteinn brought him to Chula Vista for a training camp in 2014. I remember him turning up, and Mac Wilkins greeted him and laughed and said, "What in the hell happened to Daniel? Who is this guy, and where did Daniel go?"

He was moving really well that spring, but when we went to the Irvine meet the conditions were not good. The ring was on the infield, which is nice, but there were no trees for shade and no wind to speak of, so all of us were suffering in the heat. Everyone was struggling. Nick Percy was there. Simon. Leif Arrhenius. None of them threw very well. But then Daniel gets in and hits his best technical throw ever to that point—it's actually still one of the best in terms of technique of his entire career.

On the YouTube video, you can hear Vésteinn shouting "Yeah! Yeah! Yeah!" before Daniel delivers the disc. That's how good he looked in the ring. It was 66.89m, an amazing throw, the coming together of everything they had worked on. 99

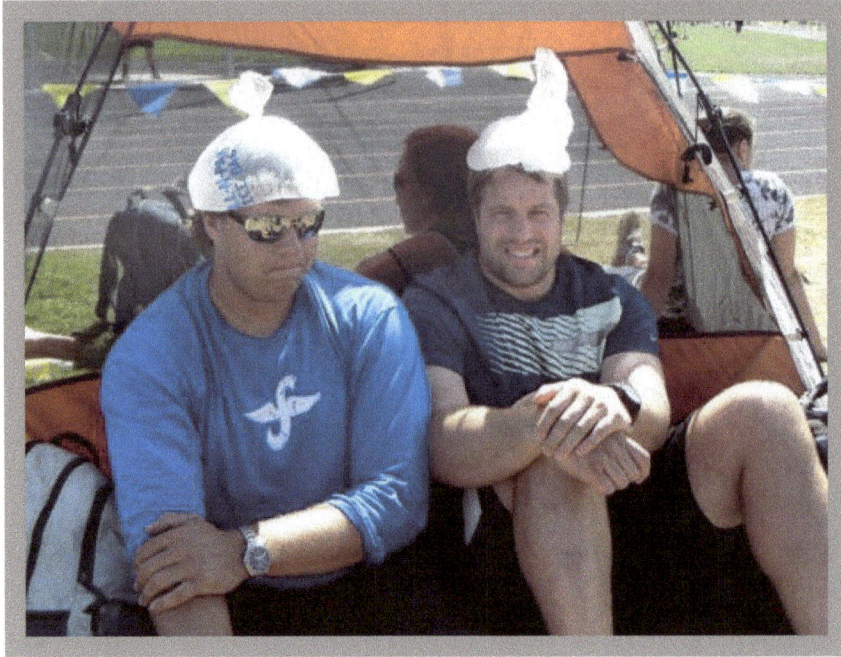

It was so hot in Irvine in 2014, so hot. But there Daniel made his breakthrough. Here sitting and waiting for the meet with Märt Israel.

At the time, 66.89m was the best throw in the world. It changed Daniel's life and almost ended his career.

I say it changed his life because up to that point, he had received no attention whatsoever for his throwing. He had never been interviewed, never been contacted by a journalist. But the day he threw 66.89m, three reporters from Sweden called saying they wanted to come to San Diego to meet him. And before the summer was over, approximately one hundred journalists from all over the world reached out to him— all because of the 66.89m throw.

And Daniel did not know how to react. For him, being a professional thrower was already hard enough when nobody was paying attention. Now the spotlight was turned on him, and for the first time he had to deal with something that for him was even worse than the loneliness and seriousness this life required: Expectations.

You see, the journalists were not just calling to ask him how he managed to throw 66.89m. They also wanted to know if he was planning on winning the European Championships later that summer.

" It was so hot that day. Before the discus comp, we were all hiding under a tree somewhere thinking we might die. When the competition started, I threw around 55 meters and remember feeling like that was a pretty amazing performance in those conditions. Then Daniel steps in and drops a 66-meter bomb on a day when all of us were like, "How are we even breathing in this?" We all started screaming like crazy, except for Shaun Pickering who was sitting next to the cage filming with an ice bag melting on his head. "

What those journalists did not understand was that Daniel had almost no chance of winning at the European Championships. Just making the final would be a big step for him.

And that is nothing against Daniel. I told him in 2011 he could be the best discus thrower in the world someday, and in 2014 I still believed it. But there is a big difference between throwing 66.89m at a fun little meet in Irvine, California, and throwing it at a European Championships in a full stadium in Zurich with television cameras pointing in your face and Robert Harting talking trash to everyone.

Even Gerd, as focused as he was, struggled to make the transition from being a guy who could throw far at a low-key meet to someone who could take a medal at a major championship. In 2002, when Gerd's season's best was 66.31m, he threw 55.14m in the final of the European Championships. In 2003, when his PB improved to 67.13m, he threw 56.63m in qualification at the World Championships and did not make the final. In 2004, he reached 68.50m in June and was considered a favorite to take a medal at the Olympics in Athens. Instead, he threw 60.05m in qualification and once again did not advance.

Gerd eventually made a breakthrough at the 2005 World Championships throwing 68.57m to take the silver medal. That was the first of eleven medals he would win in international championships, which is still a record in men's discus.

Those years of disappointment were hard on Gerd, and it is to his credit that he was able to endure long enough for his mental strength to grow to match his physical abilities.

Daniel, in June of 2014, had hardly begun the process of learning to throw well under pressure. At that point, he had never competed at a major international championships at the senior level.

Niklas Arrhenius
on the 66.89m breakthrough

66 In some ways, the 66.89m throw was a great thing because it showed Daniel he could compete with the best guys in the world. But it was also tough for him to live up to the new expectations people suddenly had.

You have to understand, athletics is a popular sport in Sweden. It's probably the main sport after soccer and hockey. If I didn't throw well in a championship, it would be written up in major Swedish newspapers. I said to my dad once, "I'll bet if Christian Cantwell didn't make the final at Worlds, not one paper in America would write about him." But Sweden is a small country, and they do write about you.

So, it was hard for Daniel for a while, because he hated the pressure and the idea of disappointing the people of Sweden. 99

And think of who he was competing against. By the summer of 2014, Gerd had thrown 66.89m or better more than one hundred times. He was a World and

Olympic champion. So was Robert Harting. Piotr Malachowski had won a European Championships and finished second at a Worlds and Olympics. All those guys had PBs over seventy meters and all had thrown over sixty-eight meters on the big stage. Daniel had thrown 66.89m once in his life at the Steve Scott Invitational in Irvine, California.

So, I was not thinking about Daniel winning the European Championships. But after being asked about it over and over, it was impossible for Daniel not to think about it, and this was very hard on him. Daniel is an extremely nice guy, and he hates disappointing people. It was clear from the questions he was being asked in the weeks after his big throw that a lot of people expected him to medal—maybe even win—in Zurich, and this made him very uncomfortable.

Arwid Koskinen
on the 66.89m throw

“ When he threw 66.89m, it was hard for me and his other friends to imagine he was so good, that he had increased so much so fast. It was a shock for us. We hadn't seen him in training much since he started with Vésteinn, and Daniel doesn't really talk about his training outside of the gym. When he's not training, he wants to have fun and play video games. Nerds like me, we talk about result, result, result, and Daniel will be like, "Come on, guys. Let's talk about something else." So, we didn't see it coming.

It was a big media thing in Sweden when he made that throw, and everyone put pressure on him. After he didn't make the final at the European Championships, they said it was a fiasco, but we knew the future was for him. ”

When Daniel went 66.89m, the dad eased off a bit and accepted Vésteinn's plan. That big throw was a massive breakthrough, but the downside was it brought attention on Daniel that he was not used to and really didn't like. But it was a big story in Sweden. Basically, two years of working with Vésteinn, and Daniel suddenly leads the world. Three journalists came to California that week to interview him. Before that, it was just fun, just Daniel doing what he was doing. But the attention brought with it big pressure. He started to feel like all of Sweden was expecting him to perform, and he's such a nice guy he couldn't stand the idea of letting people down. He told me he was worried about "disappointing the King of Sweden." After that breakthrough throw, he struggled most in competitions like the European Championships where he wore the yellow vest.

It was a treacherous situation for us both, but I decided that the best way to help him get past his insecurity and get him ready to deal with the kind of pressure a top thrower must face was to throw him into the deep end of the media pool in Zurich.

I was in charge of screening the media requests for Daniel at the European Championships, and I said yes to every one of them including for a documentary film crew which would follow him everywhere.

When Daniel asked me why I did this, I used the Swedish soccer star Zlatan Ibrahimović as an example.

"Do you think Zlatan Ibrahimović is afraid of cameras?" I asked him.

"No."

"But you are afraid of cameras?"

"Yes."

"Then we will use this Championships to get you over your fear."

And we did. The documentary crew followed him at practice, on the bus, and at meals. Another Swedish coach came to me and said I was crazy to let all those people have access to Daniel, but I was confident that exposing Daniel to a media swarm in Zurich would prepare him for the future.

Daniel ended up throwing 59.01m in qualification and did not advance to the final. Of course, some in the Swedish press described his performance as a disaster, but that is not how I viewed it. To me, he gained valuable experience in Zurich which would help him later in his career.

This would prove true in the long run, but Daniel's struggles with self-doubt were just beginning.

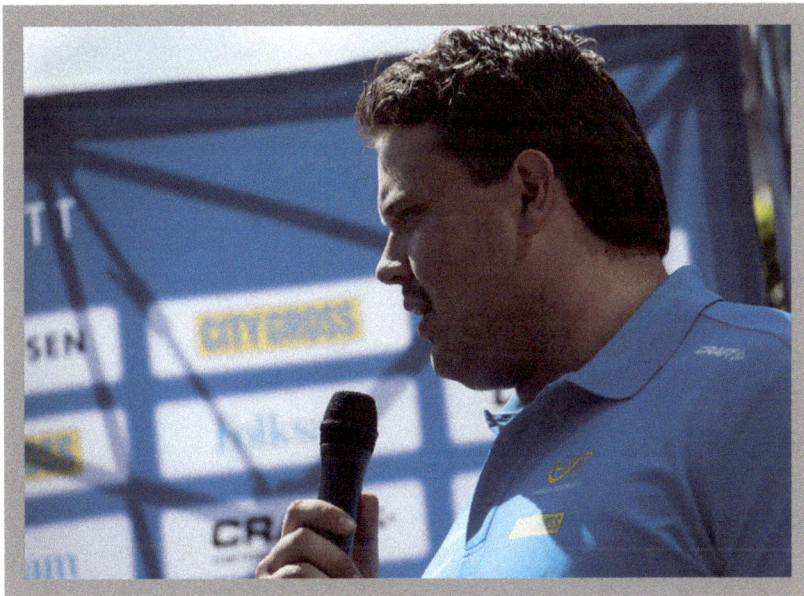

Photo courtesy of Vésteinn Hafsteinsson

Early in his career, Daniel was not comfortable talking to the media. Over time, though, he became quite good at it.

Gerd Kanter
on throwing in big competitions

" Discus is one of the hardest technical events because you have rotational and linear movement combined, and if you get tight it really affects your performance. People wonder how is it possible for one throw to be 20 meters less than your last throw, but in a rhythmical event if you are not relaxed things do not work.

And when you are preparing for a World Championships or European Championships or Olympic Games, you can say, "Oh, it is just like every other competition," but that is not true because your performance in a championship can have a big effect on your funding, and on your whole career, really.

When you get to the point where you are having a good season and throwing far enough to maybe win a medal, the pressure is so big. Even if you don't show it, you feel it inside of you. It usually takes a lot of experience to learn to handle that pressure, which is why discus is an old boy's event. "

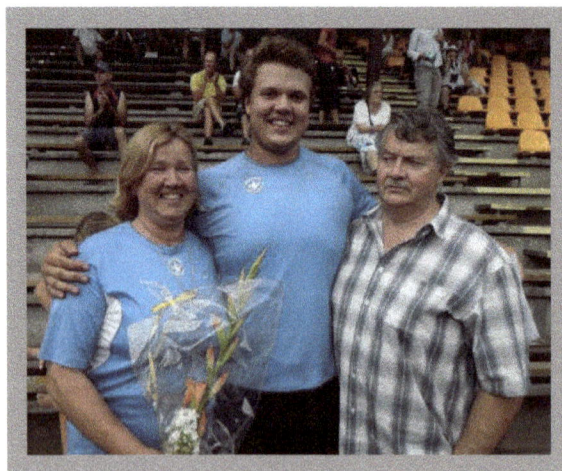

Daniel with his mother Taina and father Jan in Stockholm, Sweden

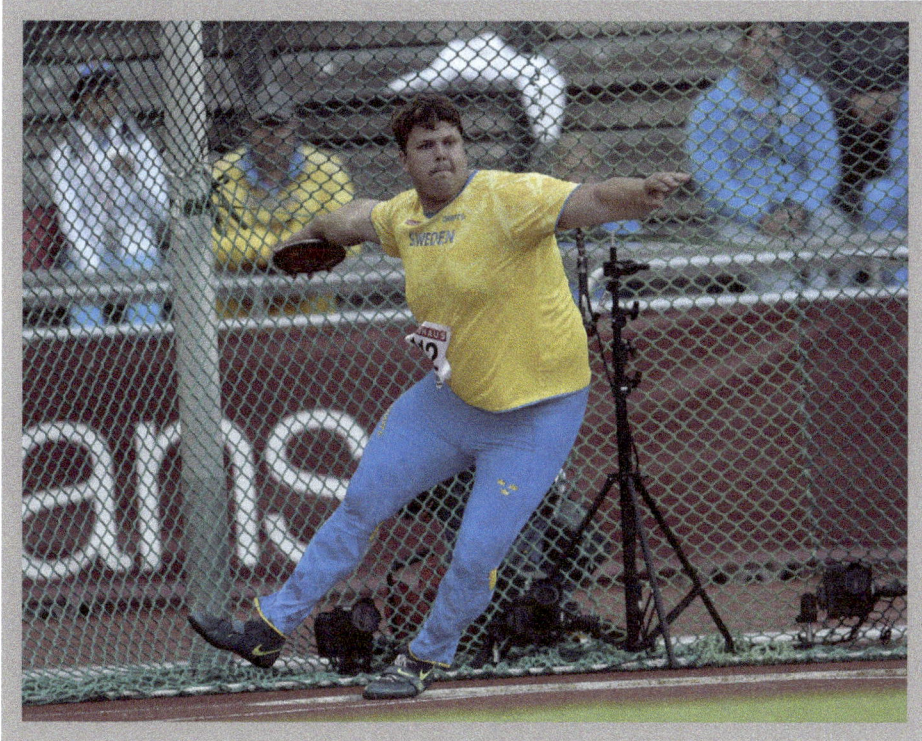

Daniel at Finnkampen 2015 in Stockholm Olympic Stadium

## 5

2015 — Hard Times
and Another Breakthrough

Prior to Daniel's big throw in California, he was a nobody in our sport. His 66.89m in Irvine made him a somebody and changed his life so much that he started to doubt he would ever be comfortable as a professional thrower.

The attention from journalists and the expectation of winning a medal at the 2014 European Championships caused Daniel great anxiety, and I could see him becoming more and more unhappy as we started training for the 2015 season.

The sense of fun and wild enthusiasm he had when he was a crazy teenager blasting discs into the cage in Stockholm was gone. Daniel became so worried about disappointing people that he could find no enjoyment in throwing.

He once again started to gain weight, which usually was a sign he was feeling down.

He never missed a training session, but an elite athlete has to take care of business in the hours between lifting and throwing sessions. They have to show up for their physio appointments, they have to eat right, and they have to get plenty of sleep. In many ways, it is a boring life, but this is the only way to become a champion, and I knew Daniel would never reach his potential if he could not behave like a professional.

This was the start of a very difficult period for Daniel, for me, and for our entire group. The fact that he came through and became a World and Olympic champion and the person he is today is remarkable. It is one of the things which makes me happiest when I look back at my coaching career.

Shaun Pickering
on Daniel's struggles in 2015

66 Daniel was not in a great place mentally during the winter of 2014-2015. He came back to Växjö out of shape after spending the holidays with his family and friends in Stockholm, which caused him to take a step back technically. We went to a training camp at Fuerteventura in the Canary Islands, and I don't think Vésteinn wanted him in the discus circle because he'd lost so much feel for the throw. Instead, they did thousands of imitations on a wide sidewalk near the beach just trying to find some rhythm. 99

But as 2015 began, there were many instances when a happy ending seemed unlikely. I started getting calls from people who knew him, including his girlfriend at the time, warning me about how unhappy Daniel was.

This was the toughest thing I ever had to deal with as a coach because I liked Daniel so much and could not bear the thought of him wasting his potential. He was always polite, always gracious. At the end of every training session, he would shake my hand and thank me for coaching him. If we were out having coffee and someone approached Daniel for a picture or autograph, he always obliged and tried to make them laugh and feel good.

A mistake I made at this time was to try to make Daniel focus by punishing him. For example, when we were planning our trip to California in the spring of 2015, I told him he could come along and train, but I would not allow him to compete in any meets.

This approach didn't work, and he became so miserable that finally in March he told me he was quitting.

"I can't do this anymore," he said. "I'll go back to Stockholm and get a job."

This was devastating news, but what could I say? If being a professional thrower made Daniel miserable, then maybe he needed to try another life. I just hoped he could find something to make him happy.

The next morning, though, he called from our training facility.

"Aren't you coming to practice?" he asked.

"I thought you fired me."

"I did," he replied. "But I changed my mind."

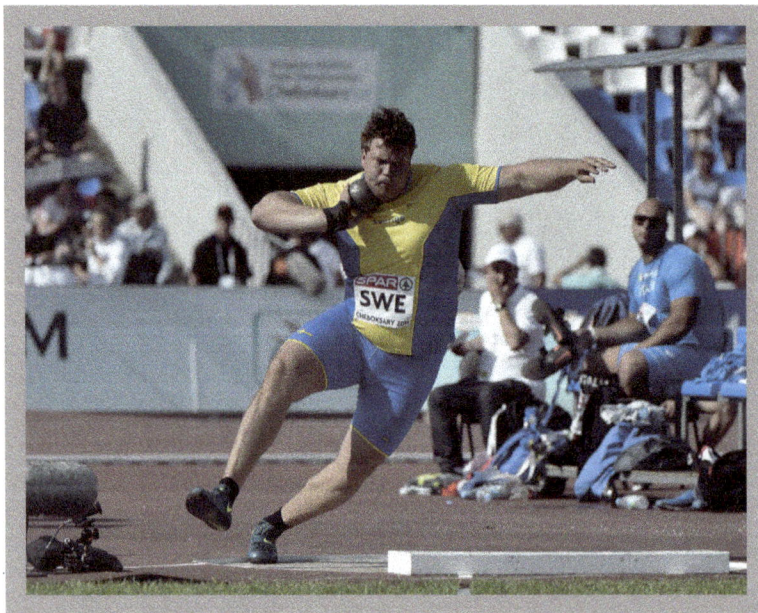

2015 European Athletics Team Championships, Cheboksary (RUS)

Daniel stayed with the group, but matters reached the point where I had to have a crisis meeting with the Swedish Athletics Federation and the Swedish Olympic Committee about his situation. To their credit, they promised to keep supporting him.

And I vowed I would, too, and do everything in my power to help him reach his potential as a thrower and as a person.

Daniel threw badly during the 2015 season and did not make the automatic qualifying distance for the World Championships. His season's best of 63.38m also left him outside of the top 32 internationally, which is where he had to be to qualify for Worlds without hitting the automatic mark.

Shaun Pickering
on Daniel's strength in 2015

" That spring, we had another camp at Chula Vista, and to cheer Daniel up, Vésteinn said to him, "I'm going to let you lift heavy and get some PRs in the weight room and have fun with that. Maybe you'll throw some shot, but we're not going to worry so much about the disc."

Daniel cleaned 200 kilos for the first time at that training camp.

I didn't see him do it, but one day I was talking to Robert Weir and he said, "Wow! Daniel can clean 200k?"

I said, "No, he doesn't really do cleans," and Robert said, "Oh yes, he does. I saw it on YouTube."

I checked, and Robert was right. "

I was coaching the Canadian shot putter Tim Nedow at the time, and I left for Korea to do a training camp with Tim prior to the Worlds, which would be held in Beijing. Then, four days after the qualification window closed, I got a call telling me that several discus throwers declined their invitation due to injury, and Daniel was now invited to the Worlds.

I called Daniel and asked, "Well, do you want to come here?"

"Yeah, I want to come," he said. "I want to come there and throw far!"

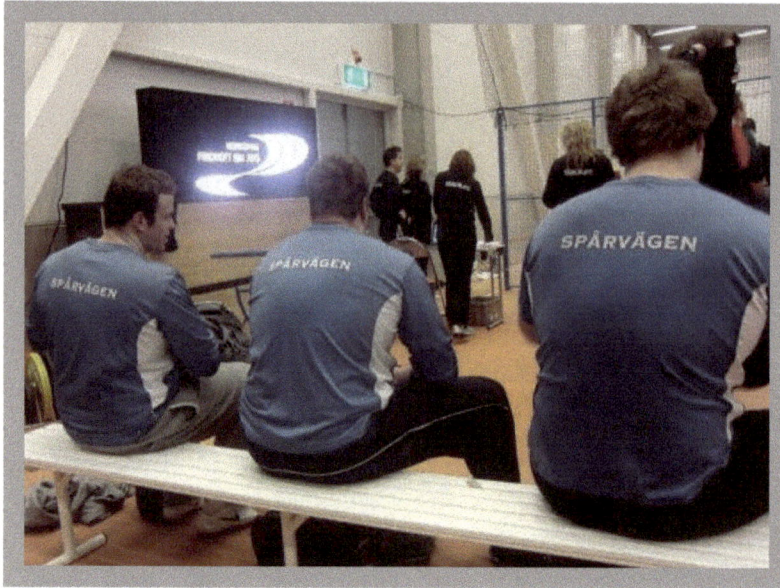

Photo courtesy of Vésteinn Hafsteinsson

Leif Arrhenius,
Nik Arrhenius and
Daniel in the Swedish
Indoor Championships
competing in Shot Put
in Norrköping, Sweden

I met him in China about a week before the competition. We were able to get in four throwing sessions, and they were the best sessions of Daniel's life so far. He was completely focused and energized. It was humid with no wind, and he threw sixty-seven meters over and over. John Godina was there as the coach for Vikas Gowda, and he couldn't believe it. We did one session at the same time as Andrius Gudžius and his coach, Vaclavas Kidykas. Afterwards, Vaclavas looked at me and said, "Daniel very good. Andrius very bad!"

Daniel had been so unstable all season I was afraid to leave him on his own while we were in Beijing. I was with him whenever we were training, but that left many hours unaccounted for, so I came up with a plan. I talked to other throwers, to Tommy Eriksson (our physiotherapist), and to Karin Torneklint (the head coach of the Swedish team), and worked it out between all of us that we would never leave Daniel alone. We literally took shifts going out with him for coffee or just hanging out in the hotel lobby.

When we got home after the Worlds, Daniel told me it had been the best trip of his life. He loved having people keep him company the whole time he was in Beijing.

And he didn't get mad at me when I admitted how I planned it all out. He thought it was a great idea.

All the socializing must have helped Daniel to relax, because he threw 62.66m in the qualification round and for the first time ever made the final at a senior international championship. Then he threw a season's best of 64.73m in the final to finish fifth.

This was a huge step forward for Daniel. As I mentioned earlier, a thrower must learn how to compete on the big stage and not just throw far with perfect conditions and no pressure. Since 2012, we entered Daniel in every damn meet we could find—around thirty each season—to get him the experience he needed to perform well in international championships.

Shaun Pickering
on the 2015 World Championships

66 Going into the 2015 World Championships, they were taking 32 athletes in each throwing event, and Daniel was ranked something like 35th, so it looked like he wouldn't be invited. But at the last minute, the Dutch decided they would only take athletes with a reasonable chance of finishing in the top eight. Their two best discus throwers, Rutger Smith and Erik Cadée, were ranked around 30th, so with them dropping out along with one or two from other countries for whatever reason, Daniel got an invite,

Vésteinn was in Korea for a pre-Worlds camp with Tim Nedow, and Daniel joined him in Beijing after that camp. Once he got there, he really got serious about training, and managed to get into good shape. Daniel ended up placing fifth, which was a massive surprise after the season he'd had.

This was a big moment for Daniel because it showed him what he could do if he focused. 99

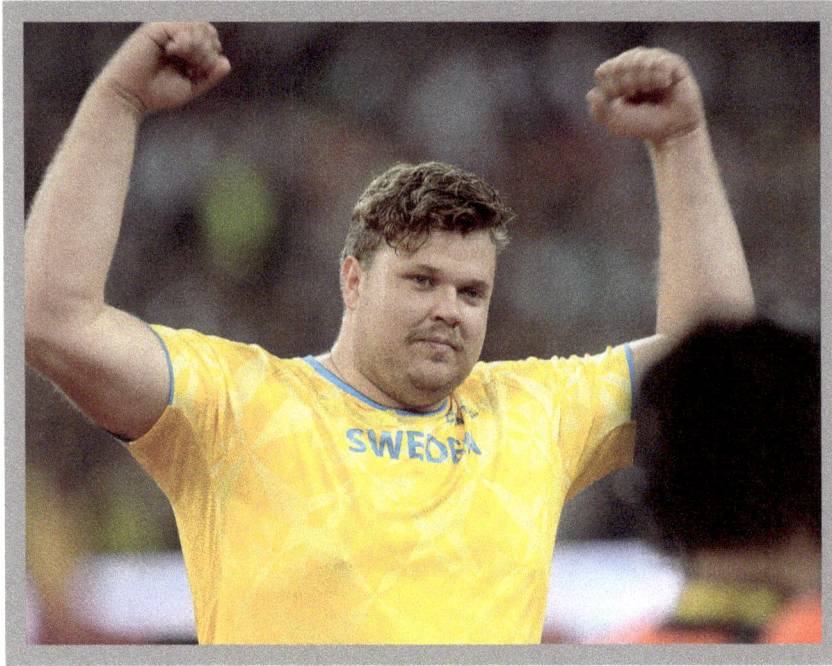

Daniel made a big breakthrough at the 2015 World Championships

In a way, his breakthrough in Beijing was a sign the plan was working. But, at the same time, I honestly do not know how Daniel threw so well there. He had been out of balance for the entire season. How was he suddenly able to get in balance for one week just before the biggest competition of his life?

And would the focus and energy Daniel showed in Beijing carry over into the next season, or would we stay on the roller coaster?

Kajsa Bergqvist
on the 2015 World Championships

" In 2014, Daniel had a big result in Irvine but then couldn't get it together at the European Championships. It was a big disappointment, and a lot of people were like, "He can't take the pressure!"

And there is a lot of pressure at the big competitions. Sometimes, you can see when an athlete is struggling mentally even before they start running, jumping or throwing. It is a certain thing in the eyes. They get a little big and wet and fishy-looking, like a blank stare. If you see someone coming into a final that way, it makes you think, "No, no, no. They are not going to perform well today."

Some athletes just get too nervous or pumped up at big moments, and they can never overcome this. But Daniel turned it around in the middle of his career to become an amazing championships thrower.

Making the final at the 2015 Worlds in Beijing and throwing a season's best there was, I think, the defining moment for him. He went from being this huge talent with possibilities to showing he really was the future of discus throwing. "

Karin Torneklint
on the 2015 World Championships

" Early on, Daniel was a very big man and also a small boy in the same body. It was hard for him that people expected him to do amazing things when he was still young and not so secure in his technique. Because he threw 70 meters sometimes people thought he should do it every time, which is tough to do—especially in a championships—until your technique becomes very stable.

For the 2015 World Championships, he was very late to get an invitation. I called him from the airport and told him, "Now I have a place for you. Will you come?"

He was very happy and said, "Of course I am coming!"

He was relieved to have gotten the chance to compete in Beijing, and it was the first time I saw him look happy to be in the arena at a championship. He ended up taking fifth place, which was a very important moment in his career because then he knew he could be one of the best in the world. "

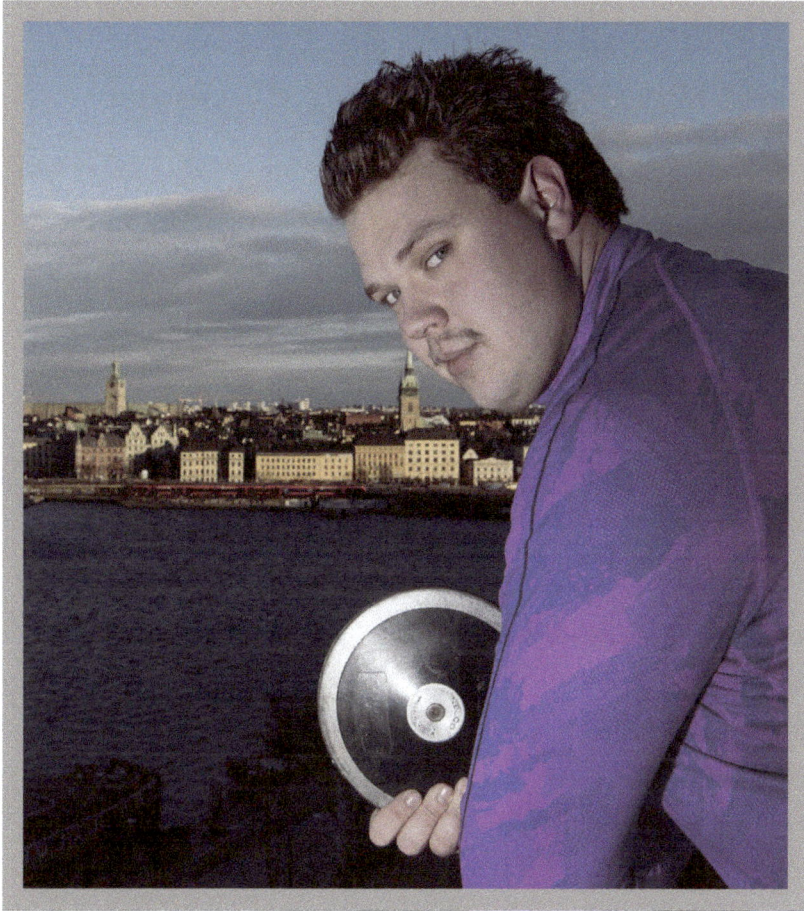

Daniel in Stockholm

6

2016 — A Hint of Things to Come

Daniel's struggles continued in the fall of 2015 and throughout the 2016 season. He had a good day at the 2016 European Championships in July, finishing fifth with a throw of 64.77m, and later in the month he threw a PB of 66.92m, but he was still unhappy, still uncertain that the life of a professional athlete was right for him. However, since he had finished fifth in Beijing and then fifth again at the Euros, there was a lot of talk about Daniel getting a medal at the Olympic Games in Rio.

I did not buy this talk.

I am a statistics guy, and the statistics from Daniel's competitions up to that point in his career indicated he rarely threw over 63 meters on his first three attempts. Sixty-three meters was the distance he would likely need to make the final in Rio, but according to my calculations he had only a 27 percent chance of reaching that mark in qualification.

Why was it important to know this? Obviously, I was not going to tell Daniel he had no chance at the Olympics. There are times when athletes defy the statistics, as Daniel had with his performance in Beijing.

But a coach has to always remain clear-eyed. By looking at the statistics instead of getting carried away with unrealistic expectations, I saw Daniel had a weakness—inconsistency in his first three attempts—which we needed to correct. Improving this would be an important part of his development. But would we have focused on this if I had believed the hype after Daniel's showing in Beijing? Maybe not.

Also, looking at the statistics and staying grounded in the real world allowed me to be a calming presence in Daniel's life, which he desperately needed. In 2014, the same reporters who hyped Daniel as a medal candidate at the European Championships, criticized him when he failed to make the final. "Disaster!" they said. "What is wrong with Daniel Ståhl?"

Karin Torneklint
on the 2016 Olympics

66 The 2016 Olympics was tough for Daniel. He was coming from a very good season, but the qualification round was early in the morning, and it was very hot weather. Also he was probably very nervous, and if you have a bad first throw and get even more stressed, it is not so easy.

And we learned that we missed some things we could have done to help him. We brought Vésteinn to Rio, but not Daniel's mental coach Henrik Gustafsson or his physio Tommy Eriksson. We realized after Rio how all three of those guys were very important to help Daniel feel well and be in a good place.

After Rio, we brought Vésteinn, Henrik, and Tommy, all the guys Daniel liked to be with, to every championships, and I think this gave him a good platform to stand on. 99

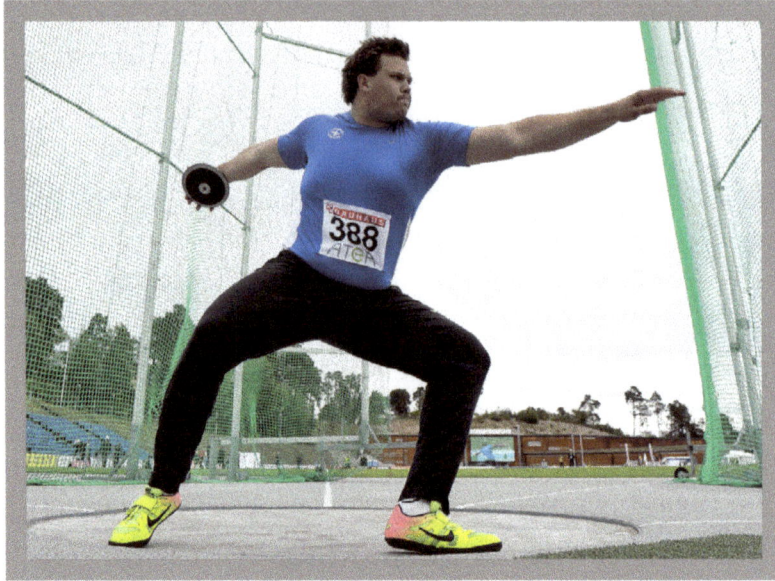

2106 was an up and down season for Daniel

But I knew nothing was "wrong" with Daniel in Zurich in 2014. He was just not yet ready to throw well on the big stage.

It was the same in Rio. Daniel threw 62.26m in qualification—not surprising based on his statistics—and did not advance to the final.

Afterwards, he knew the Swedish press was going to pummel him, and he probably thought that I would too. But because I kept a realistic view of where he was in his overall development, I was able to turn a difficult situation into something positive.

When he came out from the mixed zone after failing to qualify, I was not mad or sad. He threw far in training in the days just before the Games, and the first thing I did was to remind him of this.

"Daniel," I said. "You threw 69.60m two days ago with no wind, right?"

"Yeah. But today was terrible."

"Forget about today. You know you are in shape to throw far. In three weeks, we will go to your favorite meet on your home turf in Sollentuna and throw a PB."

"That's a great plan, man!" he replied. "And instead of watching the final tomorrow, let's go to the practice track and do our own final!"

This is something I did with Gerd Kanter at the 2004 Olympics. When I think back, it is crazy how similar Gerd and Daniel's stages of development were despite their very different personalities. Like Daniel in 2016, Gerd went into the 2004 Olympics with his head full of unrealistic expectations and knowing the press in his home country (in Gerd's case Estonia) would criticize him if he "failed."

Gerd was crushed when he did not make the final, and to lift his spirits I took him to the practice track and had him do his own "Olympic final" the next day. Gerd threw 68 meters in our private final, and while he was mad at himself for not being in the real final, this throw showed him he belonged among the best in the sport. The next year, at the 2005 World Championships in Helsinki, Gerd threw 68.57m and won the silver medal.

Daniel and I did the same thing in Rio in 2016. While the men's discus final went on inside the stadium, Daniel took six measured attempts at the practice track. All were good throws. The best was exactly 67.00m. Meanwhile, inside the stadium, Christoph Harting won the gold medal with a throw of 68.37m. It took 67.05m—just a few centimeters more

COMPARISON – Kanter vs Ståhl
THROUGH 2023

Information	GERD KANTER	DANIEL STÅHL
Personal Best	73.38m	71.86m
All Time World Best List	3rd Place	4th Place
Olympic Champion	68.82m 2008	68.90m 2021
World Champion	68.94m 2007	67.59m 2019, 71.46m 2023
All Time Top 10 Average	71.38m	71.27m
One Season Top 10 Average	69.98m	69.94m
Age, First Medal	26 Years of Age in 2005	25 Years of Age in 2017
First Four Medals in Champs	Silver, Silver, Gold, Gold	Silver, Silver, Gold, Gold
Farthest Throw in WC, OG	68.94m Osaka WC 07	71.46m Budapest WC 2023
World Leading Throw	5 Times 2005-2009	7 Times, 2016-2022

Statistical and performance comparisons of Gerd Kanter and Daniel

Fanny Roos
on training with Daniel

" I don't remember specifically the first time I met Daniel, but I think it was when he came to train with Vésteinn in Växjö, probably in 2011. I was just a shy schoolgirl then, but I remember seeing Daniel and Vésteinn and his group training in the old gym there.

I went on a training camp with them in 2015, then in 2016, I called Vésteinn to ask if he would be my coach. I was so nervous! I wrote down on paper everything I planned to say to Vésteinn on that call, and after we talked, he agreed to start working with me.

In the fall of 2016, I started training full time with the group, and I knew right away that Daniel would be nice to work with. He is a fun guy who spreads a lot of good energy, which has been really good for me. Seeing him and Simon and the other boys lifting heavy weights motivated me so much, and they have always been nice to me and supportive of me. They helped me a lot to have the career I've had. "

than what Daniel threw in our session—to win bronze. As with Gerd in 2004, this result made Daniel more confident he could compete with the top guys.

"Coach," he said afterwards. "I've only had two good training weeks in two years."

"That's right," I told him, "But, at least those came right before the most important competitions."

"Yes," he continued, "but I think we need to start having more stability in our training."

"Do you really think so?" I asked, with only a little bit of sarcasm.

Three weeks later, we went to the Swedish Championships in Sollentuna. The meet record there was 64.40m, held by Ricky Bruch. During warmups, Daniel told me he

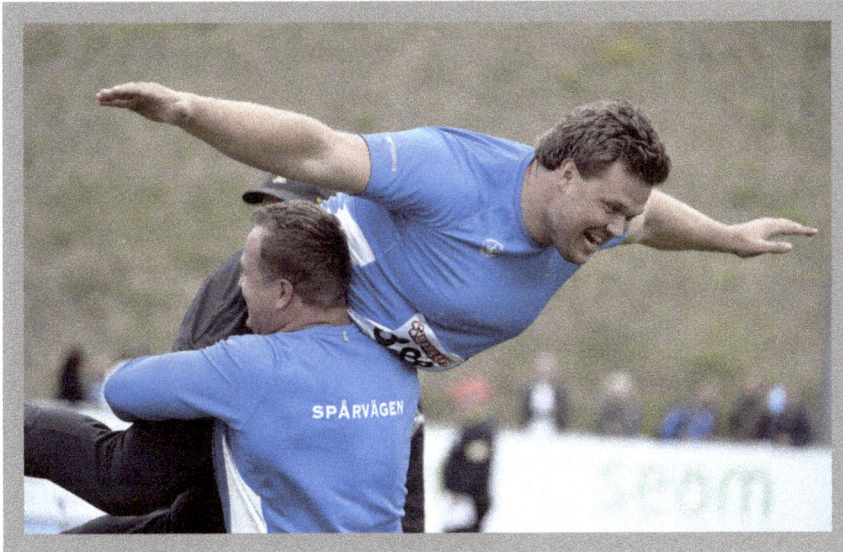

Daniel wins at Friidrotts SM 2016

was going to throw a PB, and he did: 68.72m to smash the Swedish Championships record and take the world lead.

More importantly, Daniel vowed to embrace the life of a professional thrower.

"I'm ready to go the whole way," he told me.

Two weeks later, he won the Diamond League Final in Brussels, another indication he had turned a corner in his career.

This promising finish to the 2016 season would carry over into 2017, but we were not off the roller coaster just yet.

Niklas Arrhenius
on Daniel's potential

" Over time, you could just see him getting better. Once, when we were at Chula Vista for a training camp, I watched Daniel and Simon do a drill session in the parking lot outside the Foxwood Apartments where everyone stayed, and I was really impressed with the way Daniel moved. He looked gorgeous, almost perfect. Vésteinn just stood there, hardly making any corrections. "Good job. Again. Yes. Good job. Again." I knew if Daniel could combine that technique with all his power, he'd be amazing. "

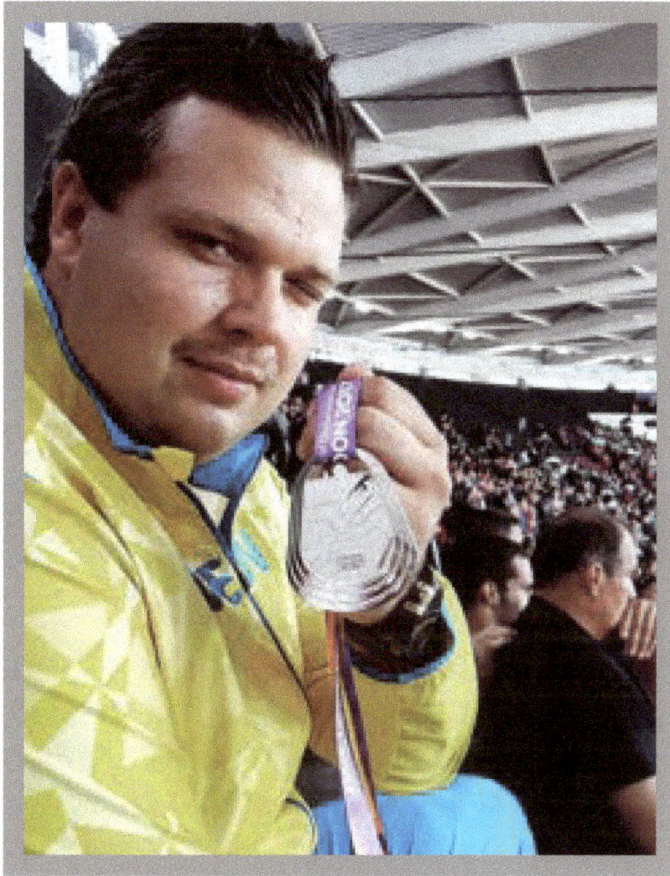

Daniel Ståhl won his first ever medal in an international championship when he threw the discus 69.19m in London at the 2017 Worlds. This was an historical moment for him as well as for Swedish Athletics and throwing in Sweden. For the first time ever, a Swedish thrower got a medal in the World Championships. At the time, it was the farthest second place throw ever in the WC in the discus.

## 7

2017— Finally, a Place on the Podium

Daniel's fifth-place finish at the 2015 World Championships was a breakthrough because it was his first success on the international stage, but his 68.72m throw in Sollentuna was an even bigger breakthrough because it convinced Daniel he had made the right choice in his life. He decided he would devote himself to becoming a great discus thrower.

We also made an adjustment in the fall of 2016 which helped a lot. For several years, Daniel lived most of the time in an apartment in Växjö. Now, we decided he would move back with his parents in Stockholm and come to Växjö for training camps every two or three weeks. This way, he could spend more time with his family and friends, which would prevent him from feeling so lonely and anxious. Daniel liked this setup, and as we prepared for the 2017 season, he was happy and stable and had a lot more energy and focus during our sessions together.

In the past, Daniel did not want to throw the discus much in the fall, but this time he did throw regularly, and his efforts paid off in February of 2017 when he achieved

66.90m at an indoor competition in Finland—a huge throw in an indoor arena where there is no wind to help the discus fly. He followed this up with some consistently excellent results when we started competing outside: 68.36m in Salinas, 68.07m in Halle, 68.06m in Oslo, 68.13m in Stockholm, and finally, 71.29m in Sollentuna at the end of June for a new Swedish record.

The 2017 World Championships would take place in London in August, and this time when people said Daniel was a medal contender, I agreed.

Look at the chart below, and you will understand why. Still using 63 meters as the mark likely needed to make an international championship final, you see that Daniel's chances had increased a lot since 2016. He now averaged 64.28m on his first throw in competition, 64.79m on his second throw, and 66.09m on his third. And his best overall throw in his top ten meets averaged 68.53m.

Statistical Comparison
of Daniel's 2016 and 2017 Performances

2017						
	Rd 1	Rd 2	Rd 3	Rd 4	Rd 5	Rd 6
Attempt average	64.28	64.79	66.09	64.00	64.97	65.17
Attempt success	68.75%	62.50%	56.25%	56.25%	73.33%	86.67%
Attempts over 63m success	37.50%	56.25%	50.00%	43.75%	53.33%	66.67%

2016						
	Rd 1	Rd 2	Rd 3	Rd 4	Rd 5	Rd 6
Attempt average	62.26	64.01	62.60	62.29	64.14	64.74
Attempt success	65.00%	60.00%	45.00%	50.00%	35.71%	78.57%
Attempts over 63m success	20.00%	45.00%	15.00%	21.43%	28.57%	64.29%

Statistics courtesy of Priit Tänava

So, for the first time in his career, Daniel could reach the final and even contend for a medal at a World Championships with an *average* throw.

There was also another factor in his favor.

Åke Ruus
on Daniel breaking the Swedish Record

" In June of 2017, Daniel competed in Sollentuna. That day, the wind did not come from the normal direction. It usually blows from the southwest, but it came from the northeast across the open water, and I thought, "Oh, the wind is perfect."

In warmups, he went 68 or 69 meters. When the competition began he hit a big throw, but there was no line at 70 meters so we had to wait for the measurement to know if it was close to Ricky Bruch's Swedish record of 71.26m. Ricky threw that in 1984 and many people considered his record unbreakable.

Then the measurement came: 71.29m. Daniel immediately sprinted 50 meters out into the field and gave the official who measured the throw a big hug. Then he threw himself on the grass and glided along the ground on his belly like a seal. Then he took a run at Niklas Arrhenius, and Niklas lifted him up, which was very impressive. "

Earlier in the season after a Diamond League meeting, Daniel came to me and said, "This was a big day. I have beaten them all now."

He was referring to the top discus throwers at the time, guys who had won championship medals like Piotr Malachowski, Robert Urbanek, Gerd, Philip Milanov, and the Harting brothers. On this day, Daniel beat Robert Harting for the first time ever, a big milestone for him.

"Great," I said to him. "What do you think that means?"

"It means I am ready for the World Championships."

I agreed, but there was another worry.

There would be a lot of press coverage of the Worlds, something I had been trying to get him used to since the 2014 European Championships. I spoke to Daniel about this when we arrived in London.

"You remember what we did in 2014?"

"Yes."

"You were afraid of the cameras then?"

"Yes."

"Can you deal with them now?"

"Yes, I can."

And he did. Daniel did not love press conferences, but he showed a lot of poise at the big one held the day we arrived in London, which included journalists from Sweden and twenty-five other countries. The Swedish coach who questioned my sanity when I allowed the documentary crew to follow Daniel at the 2014 European Championships saw how Daniel handled himself and told me, "Now, I understand what you were doing."

Going into qualification, we emphasized a single cue: push/push. Out of the back, Daniel needed to give a little push with his left leg to create horizontal velocity. Then from the power position, he needed to push with his right leg. It was that simple.

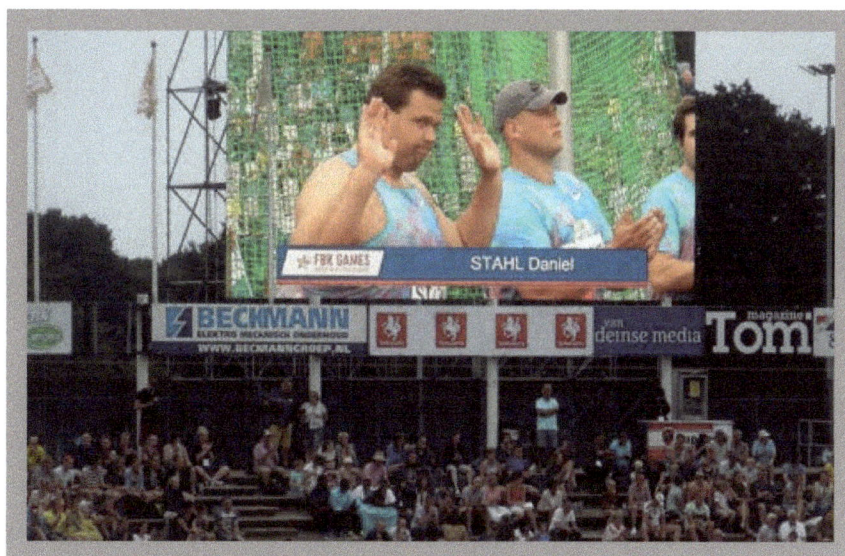

Daniel on the Jumbotron at Hengelo in 2017

" Daniel felt a lot of pressure going into the 2016 Olympics, and he was disappointed about his performance, but it seemed like he used his disappointment to get motivated. And seeing Christoph Harting—a guy Daniel's age—win might have given him some confidence as well.

And by 2017, he was getting used to competing against the best guys on the circuit. Hans Üürike and Vésteinn did a great job of getting Daniel into meets. It was really important to get him into the Diamond League so he could be around the best guys all the time. That was a big part of his development. We called in a few favors and probably got him into a few meets that he otherwise would not have been invited to. Vésteinn also asked Gerd to take Daniel under his wing at that point. Gerd became an important mentor to Daniel out on the circuit.

And Robert Harting was really kind to Daniel as well, which is funny because Robert could be difficult.

"I don't know why," Daniel would say, "but Robert is always nice to me."

I imagine Robert took a liking to Daniel because he was so fun to be around. Whatever the reason, being accepted by the guys on the circuit was a big deal for Daniel and a big part of his development. "

"If you come to me between throws," I told him, "We will not talk about anything but push/push. So, get in there, rock and roll, and remember no matter what happens, the sun will come out tomorrow and we will go back to work on Monday." We learned this mantra from our mental coach, Henrik Gustafsson, who was a huge help in getting Daniel ready to perform well at major championships.

The automatic mark in qualification was 64.50m, and on his second attempt Daniel threw 67.64m. Interestingly, 67.64m is also my personal best. It took me many years of hard work to achieve that mark, and Daniel made it look easy—but I didn't mind!

Before the final, I told my colleagues I thought Daniel would get a medal and he made me look smart by hitting 69.19m in round two. Andrius Gudžius answered right away with a throw of 69.21m, which held up for the win, and with Mason Finley taking the bronze medal at 68.03m, we now had three young giants on top of the sport of discus throwing. Gudžius, at 1.99m (6'6") and 136 kilograms (300 pounds), was the smallest of the three medalists!

It was a historic day for Daniel. He was happy and relieved and proud, and I was proud of him as well. His 69.19m was farther than Gerd ever threw in an international championship, and it made Daniel the first Swedish thrower to win a medal at the Worlds.

Daniel's performance in London also affirmed something I had been thinking regarding his weight. When he made his breakthrough throw of 66.89m in 2014, he had been following his diet carefully. After that, his weight fluctuated by as much as thirty kilos, depending on how he was feeling. Over the winter of 2016-2017, I decided to do an

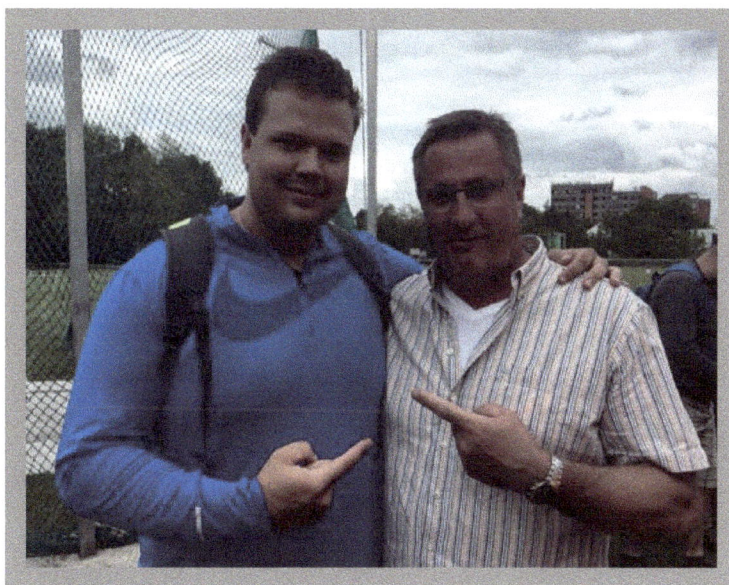

Daniel with Juergen Schult

Hans Üürike
on the 2017 season

" In 2017, Daniel had an impressive season. He went over 70 meters for the first time and got Diamond League wins in Oslo and London. This put him on the map where everyone said, "Well, he will win medals this season."

I remember the Swedish Athletics press event two days before the qualification round at the Worlds in London. Daniel was getting questions from all kinds of reporters and when he saw me, he said, "Hey Hans, come to talk to me!"

It turned out he just wanted a break where people could not ask him stupid questions, so I just stood there blocking journalists for him. I could see the Swedish media was making him nervous. Daniel is a simple guy from Stockholm who just enjoys lifting and throwing, but the rest of it... no. "

experiment and not worry so much about keeping his bodyweight in a similar range as Gerd, Robert Harting, and Virgilijus Alekna. Instead, we would accentuate Daniel's strength—literally—and he would be the biggest, strongest discus thrower ever. This helped ease some of the strain on him from always having to worry about his diet.

I still got worried though, when Daniel seemed to gain a bunch of weight just before Worlds.

I knew Daniel was in shape to take a medal if we could just stay on course for a few more days. But in the past, as I've explained, a sudden weight gain often meant he was unhappy, and I worried he had lost his focus and his confidence at the worst possible time.

I could not sleep because of thinking about this, but Henrik Gustafsson told me it was too close to the Worlds to bring up any negative issues with Daniel.

"We just have to let it go," he said, "and pray that it will be okay."

Shaun Pickering
on the 2017 World Championships

" When Daniel took the silver medal in London, it was the first time a Swedish thrower medaled at a Worlds, and Daniel was really happy about that. He didn't mind that Gudzius beat him. Daniel threw 69.19m, farther than Gerd ever threw in a major championship, which gave him a great sense of accomplishment.

World Athletics did a biomechanical study of the discus event in London, and showed the guys who finished at the top, Daniel included, all had the highest speed of release. We talked about possibly having Daniel get lighter so he could move even faster, but Vésteinn realized what separated Daniel from everyone else was he had nearly the same speed of release as the other top guys while being significantly larger than most of them. So, rather than compromise Daniel's advantages, which were his size and strength, Vésteinn decided to let him stay a little heavier. "

The only thing I did was to ask Daniel, a couple of days before qualification, "Are you feeling good?"

"Yeah," he said. "I'm feeling really good."

Then, he went out and threw 69.19m and took the silver medal.

The day after the final, we were sitting down having some coffee and I finally asked him about it.

"Daniel, you gained some weight this past week?"

"Yeah. Was that bothering you?"

"A bit."

He apologized for having worried me, then explained he had been feeling really good in the days before London and was throwing really far in training, so he rewarded himself by eating whatever he liked all week.

During our conversation over coffee that day in London, he promised to drop the excess weight. "It will only take a few days," he assured me.

But I had a different idea.

"Daniel," I said, "you threw 69.19m at at this size, right? So maybe this is your new competition weight."

As I mentioned, prior to Daniel, Gudžius, and Finley, the best discus throwers in the world generally weighed around 130 kilos, which is around what Daniel weighed when he hit 66.89m in 2014. The way he moved on the 66.89m throw seemed to confirm that 130 kilos was his ideal weight.

But watching a much heavier Daniel throw 69.19m in London, I decided it was finally time to stop trying to make him fit the mold of what great discus throwers used to look

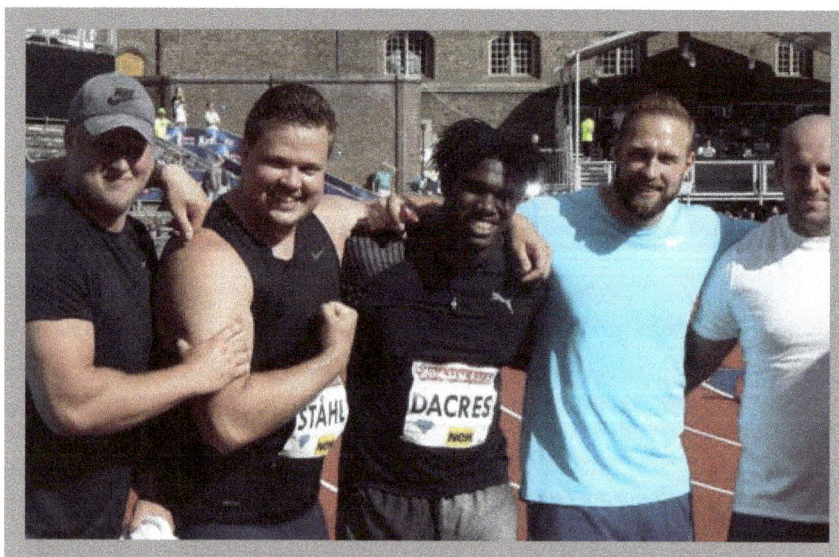

Andrius Gudžius, Daniel, Fedrick Dacres, Robert Harting, and Piotr Malachowski at Stockholm DL meet in 2017

like. We would still work to keep him fit and healthy, but we would accept the fact that Daniel was simply bigger than most other athletes.

After we made this decision, he was happier and the huge fluctuations in his weight stopped.

Also, I must point out that once again, Daniel was following the path of Gerd Kanter by winning a World Championships silver as his first international medal. And, like Gerd, Daniel had developed a rivalry with a Lithuanian. In his time, Gerd had to knock Virgilijus Alekna off the top of the ladder, and now Daniel would have to do the same with Gudžius.

That rivalry would carry over into 2018, a year which would bring more triumphs and another reckoning with the doubts Daniel had fought so hard to overcome.

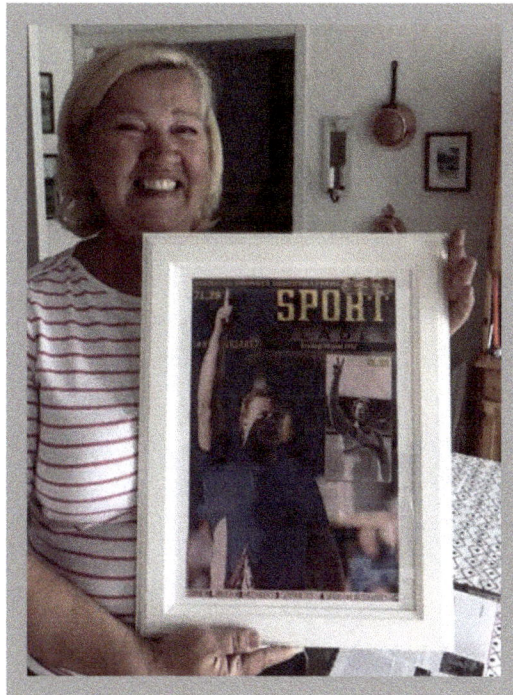

A happy mom after Daniel threw 71.29m to break the Swedish record in 2017.

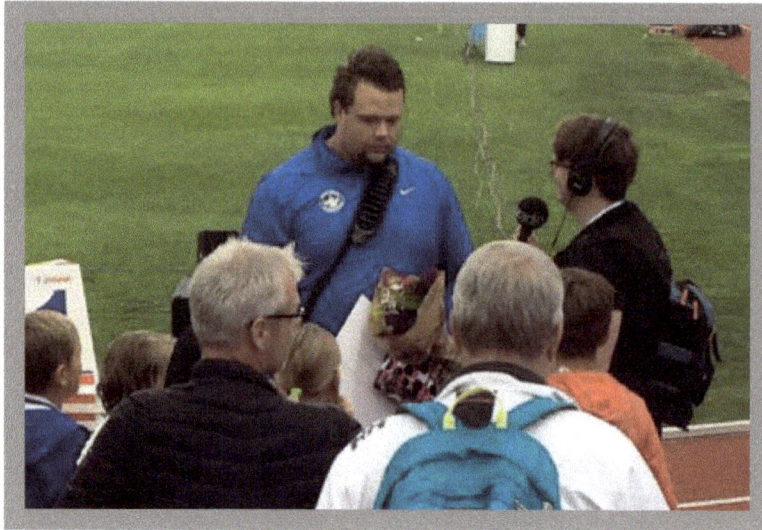

The fans are everywhere

Arwid Koskinen
on the 2017 World Championships

" I was in London for the Worlds because my girlfriend, Michaela Meijer, was competing in the pole vault. Before the qualification, Vésteinn had my favorite interview with Swedish TV where he said, "The statistics say Daniel is ready. He should take a medal." And then Daniel went and took a medal.

After the final, we met him on the stands, and it was really emotional. He was happy, but he was also trying to tell us "I am the same Daniel." He wanted to make sure we understood he was still the funny, happy guy we knew. It was important to him to keep things normal with his friends. "

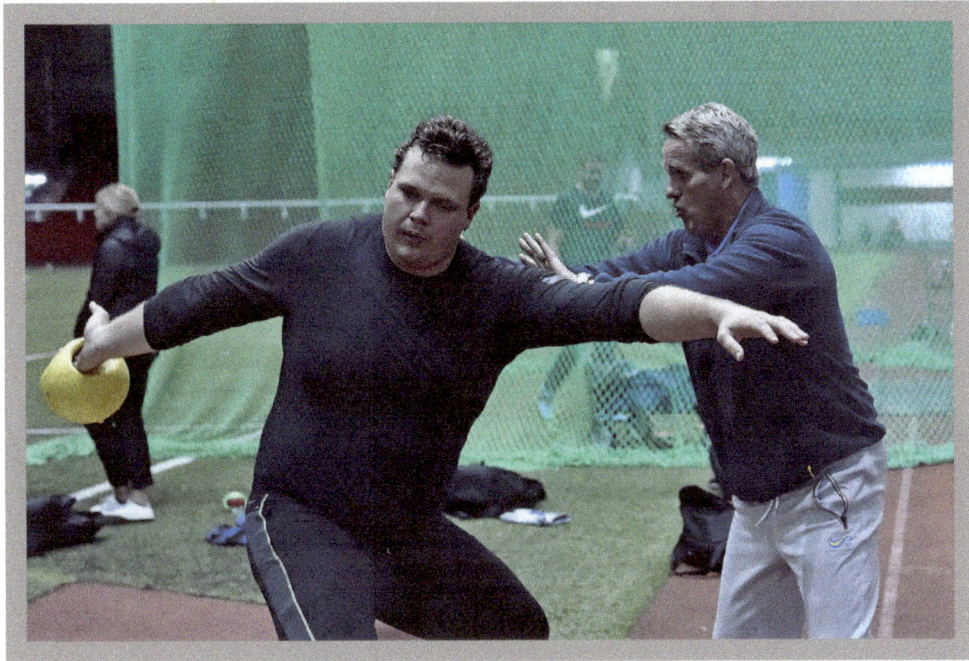

Training in Tipshallen in Växjö in 2018

8

2018 — A Turning Point

As we prepared for the 2018 season, Daniel did not train with the same passion as in 2017. It is not unusual for an athlete to feel a little tired or a little satisfied after making a big breakthrough like Daniel did in London, but with him there was still the issue of dealing with expectations. He was celebrated in Sweden for taking the silver medal at the Worlds, but it was clear that in the future he'd be expected to do even better. With a European Championships in 2018, another Worlds in 2019, and then the Olympic Games in 2020, there would be plenty of opportunities to win gold—or to fail and make everyone disappointed in him.

Daniel felt a lot of pressure from this, and I think he sometimes still regretted ever leaving Stockholm and embarking on this journey with me.

He began feeling lonely again whenever he spent time in Växjö and lost his focus. He also lost his timing in the ring, and his 2018 season was not as successful as 2017 had been.

He started off well, throwing 66.81m at the European Winter Throwing Cup in Portugal and 68.03m at a meet in Chula Vista.

But he was up and down all summer and went into the 2018 European Championships in Berlin with a top-ten average of 67.93m—half a meter less than in 2017.

I still liked Daniel's chances of taking a medal though, and thought it would once again come down to him against Gudžius. Gerd Kanter and Robert Harting were two all-time greats competing in their last international championships, but both were past the point where they could challenge Daniel if he had just an average day. Same for Piotr Małachowski. Christoph Harting was the defending Olympic champion and Berlin was his home turf, but he had struggled a lot with injuries. Of the young guys, Lukas Weißhaidinger of Austria was an up-and-comer but probably not ready to take on Daniel and Gudžius.

Despite his inconsistency, this was the first championship where Daniel and I did not talk at all about the qualification round. As I've said, it usually takes around 63 meters to advance to the final, and by 2018 Daniel could throw that far on his worst day.

He had also gotten comfortable with the slow pace of qualification rounds, which many throwers find unnerving until they get used to it. In a normal competition, a Diamond League meeting for example, there are only eight or nine discus throwers, so things move along quickly, and the athletes are not left with much time to think (or overthink) between throws. At major championships, however, there historically have been anywhere from 30-40 throwers divided into two groups for qualification. The athletes report to a warmup area outside the stadium, then are taken inside and held in a call room for an extended period, often 30 minutes or more. Once they are escorted to the infield, they receive two warmup throws with sometimes 10-15 minutes between each. Once the competition starts, each athlete has three throws to reach the automatic qualifying mark or put themselves in the top twelve. This should be easy for the best guys, but if your first throw is bad you have a long time to wait before your second. If that one is also bad, you have another long wait during which it is only natural to start thinking about how embarrassing it would be to not make the final. And once the negative thoughts start coming, it is difficult to make them stop. I have seen this many times in my career. An athlete will come over to the stands for advice between throws with their lips dry and their face white and I know it is time to pack up and get ready to go home.

This happened to Gerd during qualification rounds early in his career, so we started doing a type of practice we called "model training."

During the summer of 2005 we began putting Gerd through pretend qualification rounds at our training facility. This helped him a lot, so we did the same thing with Daniel between 2014 and 2017. At first, he struggled in our make-believe qualification rounds, but he got much better over the years, and by the 2018 Europeans I knew he would have no trouble advancing to the final.

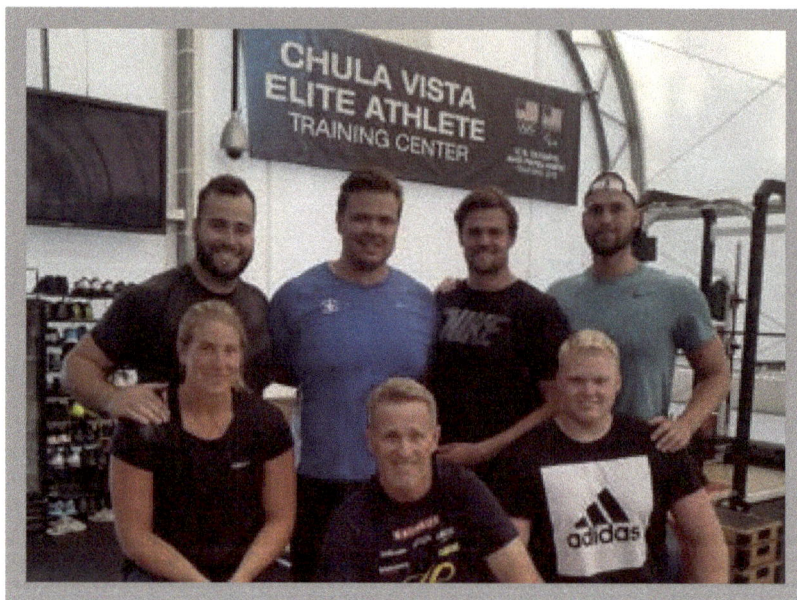

Fanny, Vésteinn, Marcus, Mesud Pezer, Daniel, Simon and Jakob Gardenkrans in Chula Vista in 2018

Daniel showed my confidence in him was warranted when he hit 67.07m—well beyond the 64.00m automatic qualifying mark—on his first attempt in qualification in Berlin.

Gudžius, on the other hand, struggled. He opened with 60.49m, then fouled before finally advancing with a throw of 64.30m.

In the final the next day, Daniel fouled his first throw, then hit 68.02m in the second round, which was far enough to just about guarantee a medal.

Then a frustrating thing happened.

Gerd Kanter
on preparing for a Championships

"In 2004, I threw 68.50m in June but ended up throwing only 60.05m in the Olympic qualification, which was not enough to make the final. Vésteinn and I knew we had to make a change, so we came up with a kind of training where we simulated the procedures used at a qualification round. We'd designate a spot at our training facility and pretend it was the call room like they have at major championships. I would sit there for a long time, just like at a Worlds or Olympics, then take only two "warmup" throws with a ten-minute wait in between, also just like at a Worlds or Olympics. Then I would have three attempts to reach 64.50m, which was around the automatic qualifying distance at most championships. Between each attempt, I would wait for twenty minutes, again just like at a major championship. The wait between throws can be very difficult. In a normal training session, if you make a bad throw you just step back into the ring and try to fix it. At a championship, you must sit there for all that time trying to stay in the moment and not overthink your next attempt. It's not easy!

During the summer of 2005, we probably did ten of those practice qualifications, and I failed in at least half of them. But I felt much better prepared for the qualification round at the Worlds in Helsinki. I threw 65.76m to advance, then 68.57m in the final to take the silver medal. That was my big breakthrough, but it took a lot of trying and a lot of failing to get there."

The head judge thought Daniel might have touched down with his heel over the front of the ring on the 68.02m throw, which would make it a foul. He checked the video, and the replay seemed to confirm his suspicions, so he nullified the throw. Daniel was now sitting on two fouls with only one more chance to move into the top eight and stay alive for rounds four, five, and six.

I was very proud of the way Daniel responded. Having a big throw disallowed in the middle of a championship final could easily have unnerved him, but he calmly walked over to the railing and said, "No big deal, I'll just go in there and throw 64.50m on my next one."

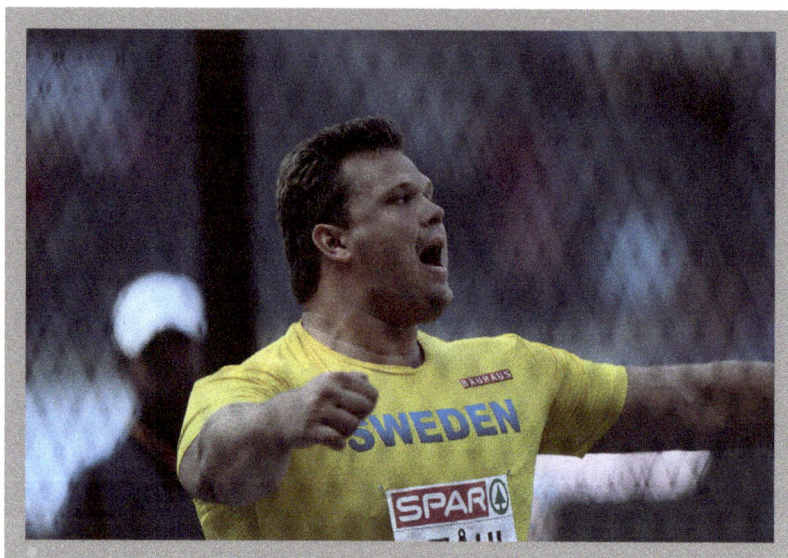

The 2018 European Championships featured another battle between Daniel and Andrius Gudžius

This was almost exactly right. He threw 64.20m, and kept his medal hopes alive. Then, in the fourth round, he reached 68.23m to take the lead.

To his credit, Gudžius jumped back into first place on his final attempt. Daniel could not respond, so once again he lost a close one to the Lithuanian, 68.46m to 68.23m.

It was still a great competition for Daniel. As I said, he took care of business on his first throw in qualification, then overcame the surprise from the field judge and once again broke 68 meters at a major championship. This showed he was maturing into a formidable competitor.

But even after medaling at two consecutive championships, Daniel was still struggling to commit himself fully to the life of the professional thrower.

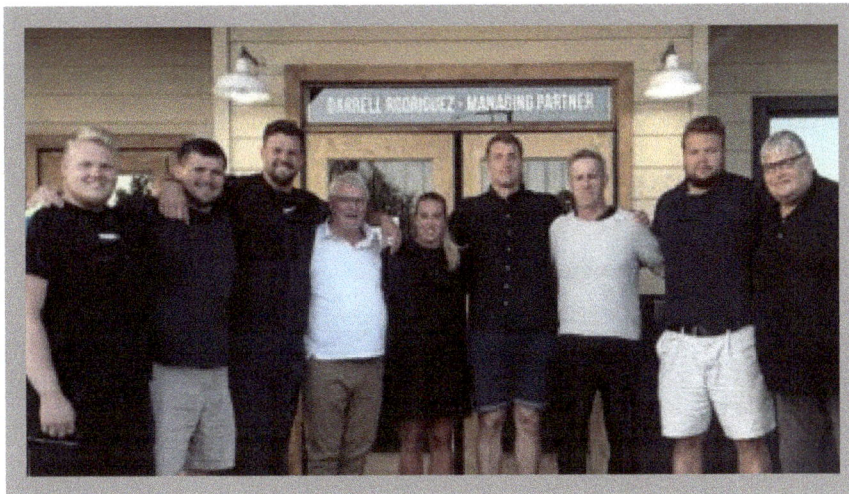

Our tradition of a steakhouse celebration for good performances in San Diego with Marcus Thomsen, Nick Percy, Simon Pettersson, Tommy Eriksson, Fanny Roos, Sven Martin Skagestad, Vésteinn, Daniel, and Shaun Pickering

Photo courtesy of Vésteinn Hafsteinsson

This was an extremely difficult moment in my coaching career. I loved Daniel and wanted him to be happy. And in the eyes of most people, Daniel had every reason to be happy. He was a World and European medalist, with the talent to maybe win the Olympics in 2020. He was immensely popular in Sweden and in his mother's home country of Finland. Wherever he went, people wanted to meet him and shake his hand and wish him well. And he got paid to throw the discus, something which he often loved doing.

But Daniel was never quite sure that he wanted to be famous, and now that he was one of the best throwers in the world, the spotlight sometimes felt too bright to him and all he wanted to do was to get away. We had some difficult times that fall, and for a while I was

"That 66.89m throw in California essentially made Daniel the face of Swedish athletics. There were a couple of Swedish journalists in the States at the time on some other assignment, and they were immediately told to drive to Chula Vista to interview Daniel. They came rolling up in a red Cadillac convertible, and Daniel was amazed like, "I'm just a guy from Stockholm and they brought this car to interview me?"

After a while, you could see how the pressure affected him. I remember watching the 2016 Olympics on television and seeing Daniel sitting alone between throws with his head down. The old Daniel would have been moving around between throws, laughing and talking to people, but the pressure was really weighing on him. He went from being this guy who was always having fun, always happy to see people, to someone who looked like he was trying to disappear.

Then, at the end of 2018 he made the decision to embrace the challenge of being the best in the world and to accept all that came with it. After that, you could see his big personality come out again."

afraid his career might be over. Finally, with lots of support from me, from our group, and from the Swedish Federation and Olympic Committee, Daniel was able to find the confidence he needed to move forward.

A year earlier, after Daniel won the silver medal in London, a fellow coach asked me, "How will he do if he ever gets completely focused?"

Now, the world would find out.

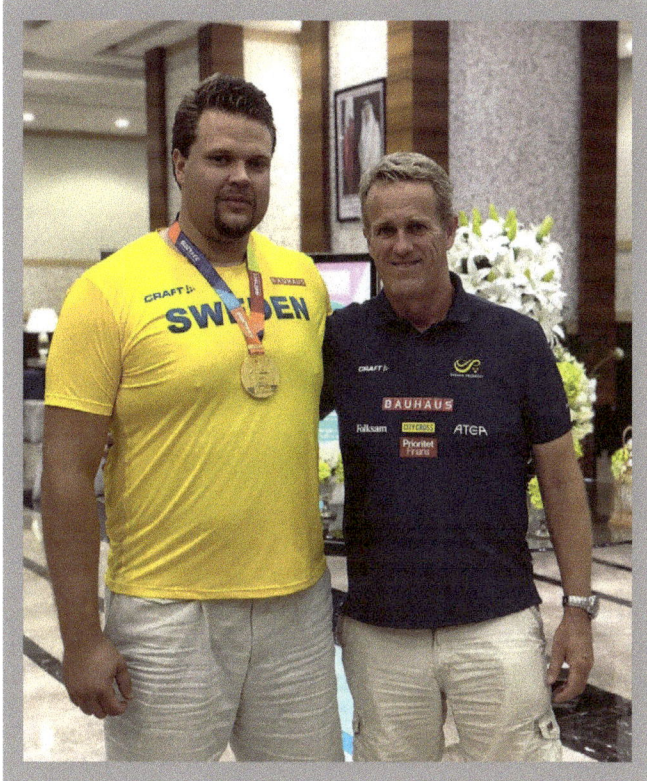

Gold medalist and coach at 2019 World Championships at Doha

2019 — On Top of the Worlds

Daniel's training went extremely well during the winter of 2018/2019. He was focused and happy and throwing very far on a regular basis. His best practice distance that winter was an excellent 68.80m in our indoor facility, which turned out to be a preview of what was to come.

Instead of doing a training camp in California in the spring, we traveled to the Gloria Training Center in Belek, Turkey, and Daniel had a great camp. In one session he threw a 72.93m training PB with a good wind. He also threw 71.05m without reverse, which showed he was in great shape and had the capacity to throw very, very far.

Daniel's first competition of the season was the Doha Diamond League meeting on May 3rd, and there he produced one of the greatest discus performances ever. His series was 69.63m, 70.49m, 70.56m, 69.54m, 69.50m, 70.32m.

Keep in mind, this was in a stadium, with no wind.

All Time Best Series Average (as of 31.10.2023)

#	Name	Country	Date	Venue	Rnd 1	Rnd 2	Rnd 3	Rnd 4	Rnd 5	Rnd 6	Series Avg
1	Virgilijus Alekna	LTU	8/3/2000	Kaunas	70.22	72.35	69.26	73.88	x	x	71.428
2	Jürgen Schult	GDR	6/6/1986	Neubrandenburg	67.20	x	x	74.08	x	p	70.640
3	Gerd Kanter	EST	9/4/2006	Helsingborg	69.46	72.30	70.43	73.38	70.51	65.88	70.327
4	Kristjan Čeh	SLO	6/16/2023	Jõhvi	68.93	x	67.92	71.70	71.19	71.86	70.320
5	Mac Wilkins	USA	4/29/1978	San José, California	70.48	70.10	x	x	x	x	70.290
6	Gerd Kanter	EST	6/28/2007	Helsingborg	70.93	68.79	x	x	70.73	70.14	70.148
7	Gerd Kanter	EST	6/25/2009	Kohila	x	69.93	x	71.64	68.03	70.92	70.130
8	Virgilijus Alekna	LTU	7/14/2008	Réthymno	67.95	70.55	x	70.86	70.76	x	70.030
9	Daniel Ståhl	SWE	5/3/2019	Doha	69.63	70.49	70.56	69.54	69.50	70.32	70.007
10	Imrich Bugár	CZE	8/26/1984	Nitra	69.66	70.24	x	x	x	x	69.950
11	Gerd Kanter	EST	4/28/2009	Chula Vista, California	x	70.84	x	69.05	x	x	69.945
12	Virgilijus Alekna	LTU	8/11/2000	Zürich	70.26	68.55	68.68	70.42	70.60	71.12	69.938
13	Daniel Ståhl	SWE	8/10/2020	Sollentuna	68.38	x	71.37	x	x	x	69.875
14	Daniel Ståhl	SWE	7/15/2019	Varberg	67.99	68.79	70.78	70.36	70.89	70.37	69.863
15	Daniel Ståhl	SWE	6/29/2019	Bottnaryd	68.76	68.83	69.71	x	71.86	x	69.790
16	Gerd Kanter	EST	5/3/2007	Salinas, California	70.52	68.02	x	x	72.02	68.50	69.765
17	Kristjan Čeh	SLO	5/5/2023	Doha	70.89	x	68.95	68.46	70.70	x	69.750
18	Virgilijus Alekna	LTU	8/23/2004	Athína	69.89	x	x	x	69.49	x	69.690
19	Luis Mariano Delís	CUB	5/21/1983	La Habana	x	68.84	69.52	x	71.06	68.74	69.540
20	Lukas Weißhaidinger	AUT	5/19/2023	Schwechat	68.36	70.68	x	x	x	x	69.520
21	Daniel Ståhl	SWE	5/30/2019	Stockholm	x	69.57	x	69.33	x	x	69.450
22	Daniel Ståhl	SWE	8/25/2019	Stockholm	69.42	69.39	x	x	x	x	69.405
23	Kristjan Čeh	SLO	5/28/2023	ar-Rabāṭ	70.07	69.38	68.26	69.10	70.32	69.20	69.388
24	Gerd Kanter	EST	5/6/2010	Chula Vista, California	68.74	69.73	69.83	69.55	68.56	69.28	69.282
25	Lars Riedel	GER	8/14/1996	Zürich	66.98	68.64	69.32	69.26	70.38	71.06	69.273
26	Mac Wilkins	USA	6/11/1976	UCLA, Westwood, Californ	68.64	68.30	69.50	69.70	70.10	69.16	69.233
27	Virgilijus Alekna	LTU	3/30/2001	Stellenbosch	70.59	66.11	x	x	70.99	x	69.230
28	Kristjan Čeh	SLO	6/26/2021	Kuortane	x	67.81	70.35	x	68.54	70.22	69.230
29	Virgilijus Alekna	LTU	6/11/2000	Tartu	68.34	70.06	68.99	70.39	68.30	x	69.216
30	Virgilijus Alekna	LTU	6/23/2004	Réthymno	68.61	69.08	70.02	67.85	70.97	68.76	69.215

Statistics courtesy of Priit Tänava

I was at home in Växjö following the live results on my computer, and after two throws I started to cry. It had been a long road since I first went to Stockholm to see this big, out-of-control kid launch discs all over the place. In the years since, he achieved some excellent results including silver medals at the World and European Championships, but along the way he lost the joy he once had in throwing. Now, the joy was back, and the world would finally see what a guy with Daniel's size and smooth moves could do.

He threw 69 meters again on May 30th in Stockholm, then again at three more competitions in June before setting a new PB of 71.86m in Bottnaryd, Sweden, at the end of the month.

Over four competitions in July, he went 68.93m, 68.77m, 70.89m, and 68.56m. He surpassed 69 meters twice in August, then won the Diamond League final in Brussels on September 9th with 68.68m.

Statistically, it was the best year in history for any discus thrower at that time. Gerd, in 2007, had the all-time best top ten average of 69.98m, but seven out of those events were throwing meets held in open fields. In 2019, Daniel's top ten average was 69.94m with nine of his best efforts coming at regular competitions inside stadiums.

After the Diamond League final, there was one more river to cross. Daniel, for the first time, would enter an international championship—in this case the Worlds in Doha—as the favorite to take the gold medal. All season, the media depicted him as being this huge, fun-loving guy who nobody could beat. This was flattering, but it meant anything less than a gold medal in Doha would be considered a failure.

2019 Best Top 10 Average: 69.94m

RESULT	MEET	LOCATION
71.86	Bottnarydskastet	Bottnaryd, SWE
70.89	Folksam Grand Prix	Varberg, SWE
70.56	Diamond League	Doha, QAT
69.94	Diamond League	Rabat, MAR
69.89	Team Championship	Malmö, SWE
69.57	Diamond League	Stockholm, SWE
69.42	Sweden vs Finland	Stockholm, SWE
69.23	Swedish Championship	Karlstad, SWE
69.12	Folksam Grand Prix	Sollentuna, SWE
68.93	Folksam Grand Prix	Karlstad, SWE

Statistics courtesy of Priit Tänava

This was a lot to deal with, especially for someone like Daniel who always worried about disappointing people. Over the years, I've seen athletes like Robert Harting and Usain Bolt who love the spotlight. Simon Pettersson is like this, also. Even though Simon is a shy person in regular life, when he walks into the stadium at an Olympics or World Championships, he is the happiest man on the planet. From the look on his face,

Åke Ruus
on Daniel at the Doha Diamond League

❝ Daniel's 2019 season began with a training camp in Turkey for three weeks, then he went directly to the Doha Diamond League meeting. Vésteinn went home after the camp in Turkey, and I went to Doha with Daniel.

We arrived the day before the competition, and it was 38 degrees Celsius (100 degrees Fahrenheit). We were at the training field, just watching the shot putters, and Daniel told me he was having trouble sitting still. He was very excited about the competition because he felt like he was in such good shape.

The next day, we talked about changing his position at the back of the ring because the cage looked a bit narrow. He did that and had an amazing series.

His first throw was 69.63m, then 70.49m and 70.56m. He got a bit tired after that, but I encouraged him to keep focused. Then he went 69.54m and 69.50m. The other throwers were just standing around watching him with big eyes. They all clapped on his final attempt, which was another 70-meter throw. ❞

you'd think it was his wedding day. It never occurs to people like Simon or Robert Harting that they might have a bad result in a big competition. They get caught up in the excitement and use it to their advantage.

Gerd was not like this. As I described above, he had to learn how to compete on the big stage. Daniel had been through the same process as Gerd, and now in Doha we would see if he was ready to handle the pressure of being the favorite.

I knew Daniel was prepared physically. He threw extremely well at our pre-camp in Rome and easily made it through qualification in Doha by throwing 67.88m—more than

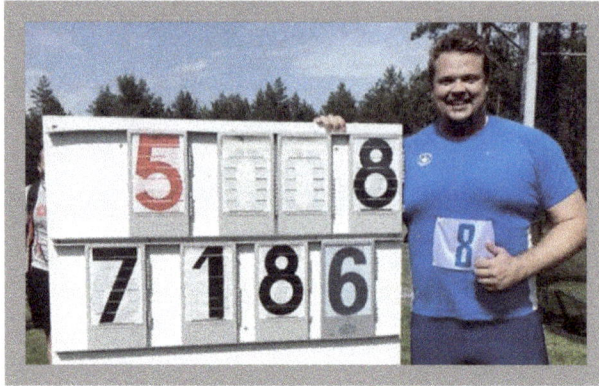

New Swedish
National Record

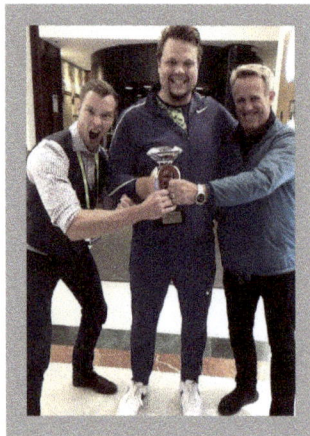

Hans Üürike with us celebrating
DL final win in 2019

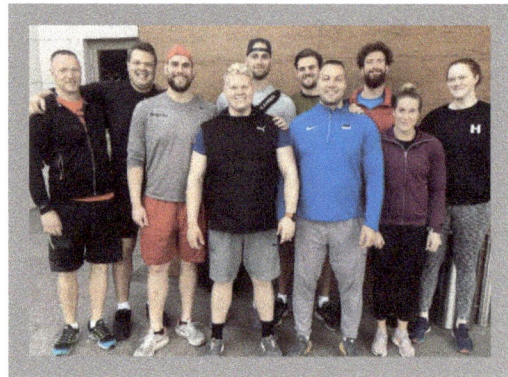

Training camp in Belek, Turkey. Rait Sinijärv, Daniel,
Viktor Gardenkrans, Marcus Thomsen, Jakob Gardenkrans,
Simon Pettersson, Kristo Galeta, Martin Kupper,
Fanny Roos and Daniella Persson

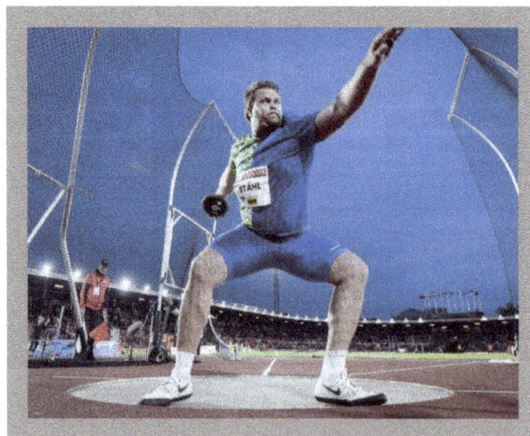

DL in Stockholm 2019
also a winner

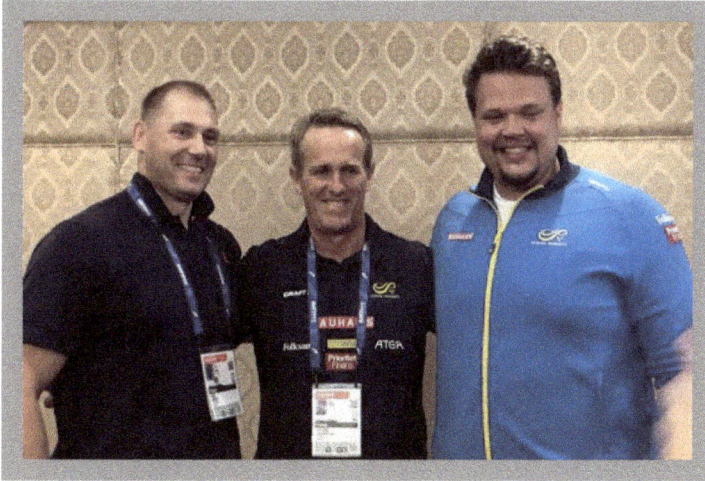

Two World Champions, Gerd won in 2007 and joined in on the celebrations with Daniel taking the title in 2019 in Doha.

two meters farther than anyone else. But I got shook up when Daniel and I sat down for a meeting with Henrik Gustafsson the night before the final.

As we were finishing, Daniel got up and said, "Well, I guess I have to win tomorrow."

This showed he was feeling the pressure. "Wanting" to win is one thing, but feeling you "have" to win means you are worried about losing. This makes it difficult to relax, have fun, and rock and roll.

Niklas Arrhenius
on Daniel's power

" I remember being at a session with Daniel where he threw 69 meters or something, and it felt like an earthquake was happening. I had been around Gerd Kanter in his prime. I threw against Virgilius Alekna, Lars Riedel, Piotr Malachowski, and Robert Harting. But I'd never had the sensation I felt watching Daniel that day. He was moving incredibly fast for a man his size, and it made me feel like nothing was impossible for him. "

> He felt a lot of pressure going into the Worlds as the big favorite and ended up having his worst performance of the year in terms of distance. It didn't help matters that the officials would not allow him to use his favorite discus at Worlds. It was an old Nelco black disc, a kind they didn't make anymore. It was just an average disc, but he liked it and used it so much that by the time of the Worlds it was pretty beaten up and they disallowed it. He ended up having to throw a fresh-out-of-the-box disc, which he did not like. He struggled and left the door open for someone to step up and challenge him, but Daniel was so dominant that year, nobody believed they could beat him.

The next day in the final, I saw the pressure was definitely bothering Daniel. He struggled the whole time with his technique and never made a smooth, rhythmical throw.

What saved us was all the years of training, of travel, of throwing anywhere, anytime, in any conditions, of making Daniel so big and strong and tough that even on a bad day he could not be beaten.

His best throw in the final was 67.59m, which was two meters below his top ten average for the season, but he got over 67 meters three times and nobody else did. The silver medal went to Fedrick Dacres, who threw 66.94m.

He was very happy afterwards, and I was extremely proud of him. When journalists asked why he didn't throw better, Daniel gave the perfect answer. "This was not about throwing far," he said. "It was about winning."

A few weeks later, Daniel gave an amazing presentation at the Swedish Sports Awards where he described me as a character from a Viking saga. Fanny and Simon told me later that he'd been working on it for weeks, going off by himself and writing down notes

Daniel's Speech

Then there is one more person that I want to thank especially. I want to do that with a quote from a man, a Viking, which is talked about in an Icelandic family saga.

He was big and strong and could handle a weapon better than any other man in Iceland.

He could chop and threw a spear as well with one hand as the other.

He could swing his sword so fast that you could see three in the air at the same time.

He could swim as a seal and in general there was no play that it was worth for anyone to try to stand against him.

He was smart and farsighted, helpful with advice and deed with his friends but as tough against his enemies.

But, the saying about him is that he loved and could kill with the same warm hand.

And his name is Vésteinn Hafsteinsson.

which he refused to show them. It turned out to be the best speech I've ever heard, and I've heard a lot of speeches! It takes poise and confidence to get up and talk in front of a packed hall with the whole country watching on television, and I've never seen anyone pull it off the way Daniel did that night.

Listening to that speech, I was extremely proud of him. He had gone to Doha carrying the weight of his country's expectations and come home a World champion. Now, there was one more hill to climb.

Arwid Koskinen
on the 2019 World Championships

" I was watching on television at my place with our friend Elias Håkansson. We heard from Vésteinn that Daniel had been throwing far in training, so we knew he had a lot in the tank, but when the final started, he looked really uncomfortable. He kept backing off on his throws, and we were like, "Okay, this is going bad." But he had so much power, he still beat everyone.

And then we saw he was going to jump the damn hurdles. That made me nervous. But we were so happy for him. Elias and I called him, and we had a nice talk. It was a huge moment. The silver in London was great, but this was a gold medal. But he was still the same Daniel. He always takes time for his friends. "

Tommy Eriksson
on the 2019 World Championships

" Daniel had so much pressure on him at the 2019 World Championships. Everyone expected him to take the gold and maybe even break the world record. And then the heat was so strong, it was hard for the big guys. I was really impressed with how Daniel handled everything.

After he won, we were in my treatment room there in the hotel and Daniel told me, "Now, a big stone has fallen from my heart." And then he started to cry from happiness. "

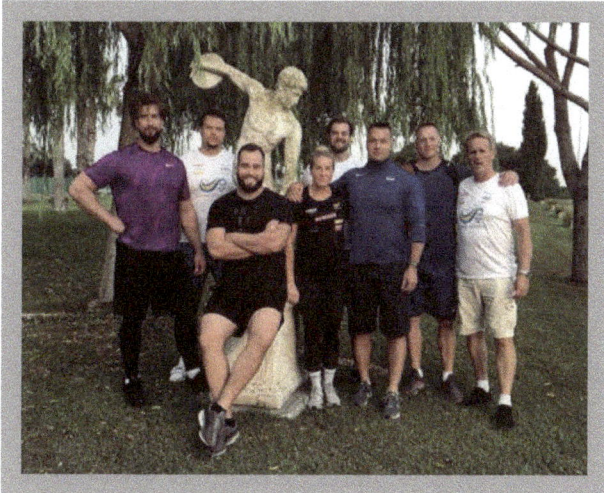

In Rome at the Ostia Training Center camp before the WC in Doha.
Martin Kupper, Daniel, Mesud Pezer, Fanny Roos, Simon Pettersson,
Kristo Galeta, Rait Sinijärv and Vésteinn

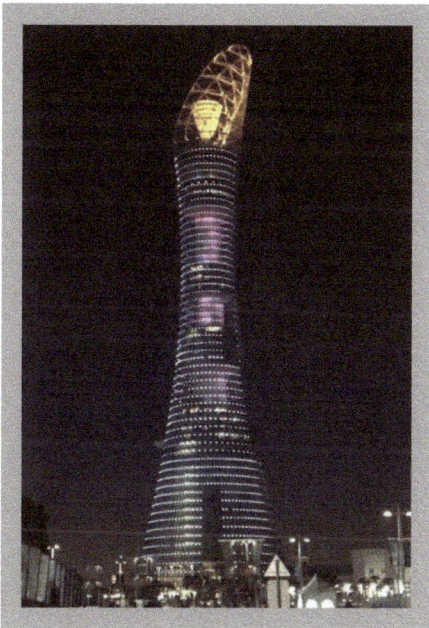

Aspire Tower, also known as The Torch Doha,
is a 300-metre-tall (980 ft) skyscraper hotel located
in the Aspire Zone complex in Doha, Qatar

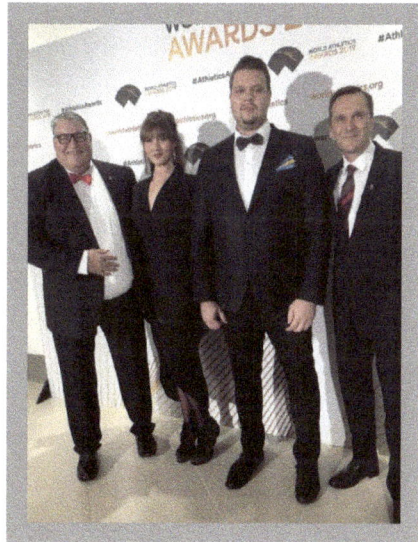

At the WA Award Ceremony in Monaco with
Shaun, Anneli Ståhl the sister of Daniel and John
Ridgeon, the General Secretary of WA.

Hans Üürike
on the 2019 World Championships

" Worlds was stressful! The weather in Doha was tough with the temperature 40-plus degrees centigrade in the shade. Yes, the stadium was air-conditioned, but the whole situation was stupid. One minute you are outside, and it is 40 degrees centigrade. Then, you get on a bus that feels like a refrigerator, and your body is shocked. You feel like, "What the hell is going on here? I need more clothes!" Then you get off the bus, and once again it is 40 degrees. Then, you go into the stadium, and you are cold again. Being there for six or seven days leading up to the qualification for sure affected the big guys. Daniel's top-ten average in 2019 was 69-high and he ended up winning at the Worlds with 67.59m. That was quite stressful to follow in the stadium. We saw the big guys were not themselves, and we worried that maybe a smaller guy throws 67 meters, and the perfect season is done. Luckily, Daniel got the deserved win. "

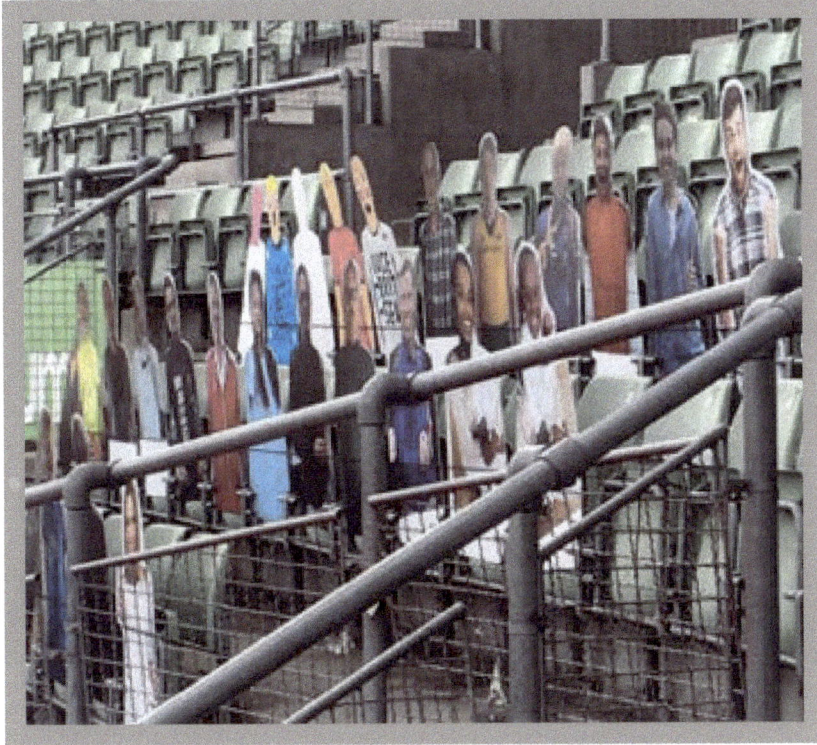

The Impossible Games in Norway. Boring meet with artificial spectators.

10

2020 — An Unexpected Interruption

After taking the gold medal at the World Championships in 2019, Daniel would again be the favorite going into the 2020 Olympics. He seemed to be at peace with this and to accept the attention which followed his success in Doha. He remained in good spirits as we trained that fall and winter, and I was optimistic he could pick up where he left off in 2019. Then Covid arrived and made 2020 a strange and difficult season.

We went to South Africa for a training camp in January, but because the virus was spreading, we were not able to make our usual trip to Leiria, Portugal, at the beginning of March. Then, just as we were about to head to California for our annual training camp at Chula Vista, the world shut down.

Soon, it was announced the 2020 Olympic Games would be postponed for a year.

I was very worried about Daniel when this happened. We were lucky because the rules in Sweden were different than in most countries. Our facility was never closed, and we did not miss a single session of training. But Daniel really enjoyed competing against the other guys on the circuit, and without having that to look forward to, I was afraid he might start feeling bored and homesick and once again lose focus.

This was also a frustrating situation because an athlete is only at their best for a limited amount of time, and the clock was ticking for Daniel. He dominated in 2019, and if the Olympics had happened in 2020 as planned, I expected him to smash everybody and take the gold. But after a year's delay, would he start to lose his edge? I didn't know.

I believe, though, that we must always make the best of our situation and focus only on what we can control without making excuses. This is something I learned from Al Oerter, the four-time Olympic champion in the discus. Al told me if there is a problem,

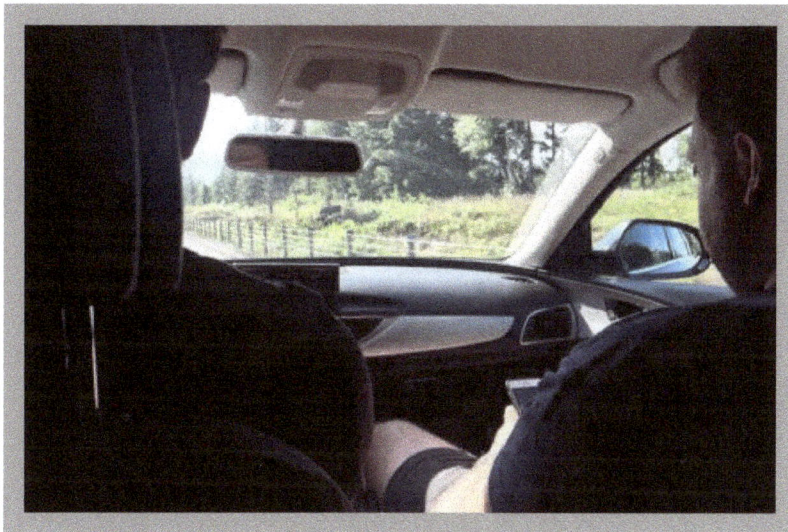

Photo courtesy of Vésteinn Hafsteinsson

On the road again, Simon driving with Daniel in the front seat and me in the back in 2021. During 2020 and 2021, it was mostly cars that were used to get to meets due to Covid.

you deal with it and do not let it turn into an excuse to perform badly or skip training. I preach this to my athletes all the time. Throwers are always complaining about silly things like bad weather at a competition. "Oh, the wind was terrible!" or "The ring was

Nick Percy
on the Covid lockdown

66 We were all on a camp in South Africa in January of 2020, and Vésteinn sat us all down and said there was something called Covid going around that might affect the European Winter Throwing Cup. There were rumors that Portugal, where the Cup is held, might shut down, and things were starting to feel a bit weird, but Vésteinn was cool as a cucumber and just kept telling us everything would be fine. During that camp, I roomed with Simon, and he got so sick he was bedridden for four or five days. Then I got sick as well. At the time, we thought that Covid was just in China and Italy, but I wonder looking back if that's what we had.

It ended up being a great camp in South Africa, and we had the whole year planned out, but the virus had other plans. 99

really slick!" My athletes know they cannot say these things to me. If they do, I will tell them to shut up and do their job and it is their fault if they did not bring the correct shoes to use on a wet ring.

After a competition a few years ago, Daniel said to me, "I know you don't want any excuses, but I threw a PB today in the shot put and it was pouring rain."

I said, "Congratulations, Daniel. That is great. But I do not care if it was raining!"

To me, this is part of being a professional. You focus on doing your job and and forget about the things you cannot control.

Dealing with a pandemic is obviously more serious than dealing with a rainy day, but I tried to apply this same philosophy throughout the 2020 season by constantly telling my athletes how lucky we were to be able to train every day when athletes from many countries could not.

I also tried to make things feel as normal as possible. We always looked forward to our time in California in the spring, but since we could not travel in 2020, I tried to replicate the training camp feel here in Växjö. We followed the normal training camp schedule and just tried to ignore the fact there were no palm trees.

And since many international competitions were canceled, we put together our own season in Sweden. In June, we received permission to hold small throwing meets with up to fifty spectators, and those meets ended up getting television coverage and bringing a lot of attention to the throws.

Hans Üürike
on the 2020 season

" Things were crazy in 2020. Everyone was in shock, wondering what the hell was going to happen. Vésteinn had planned a long time for the 2020 Games, and Daniel was clearly the best in the world at that point, but it cost him a lot of motivation when the Games were postponed. When the Olympic Games are coming, it is easy for a coach to keep up the motivation in training, but it's different when there are no championships at the end of a season. Luckily, Vésteinn is a very good psychologist.

The main question was how long Daniel could last on this high level. You just never know. You can be in top shape, then you get an injury, and you are out for two years. So, we wondered if something might happen to take away his chance to win the gold medal at the Olympics. "

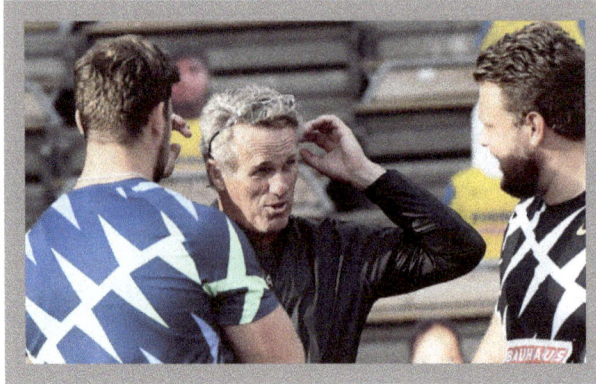

At Bauhaus DL meet
in Stockholm in 2020

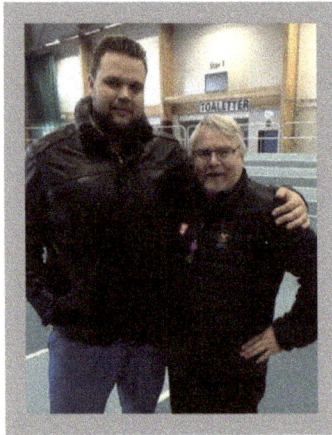

Daniel with Tommy Eriksson, our
team physiotherapist

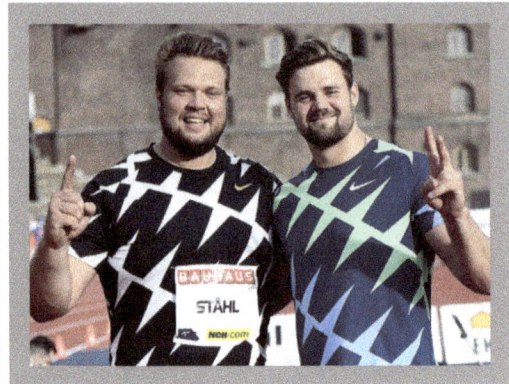

Daniel and Simon at DL meet in Stockholm

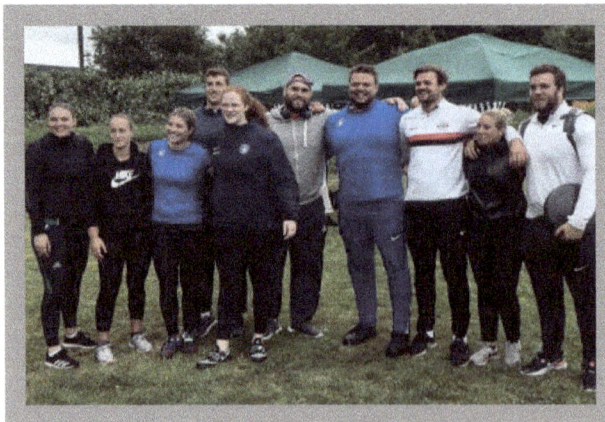

After the "Covid" meet in
Helsingborg, Sweden.
Mathilda Eriksson, Ella Andersson,
Emma Ljungberg,
Sven Martin Skagestad,
Daniella Persson, Viktor Gardenkrans,
Daniel, Simon, Fanny and
Wictor Peterson

But I was worried about Daniel the whole time. The postponement of the Olympics for sure affected his motivation, and he was not in great throwing shape when we started competing. He had a good winter in the weight room, so he was strong like a Caterpillar tractor, but his rhythm in the discus ring was off and he threw poorly (65.92m) at our first meet in Oslo on June 11th. He did even worse a few days later at a meeting in Södertälje, Sweden, where he fouled every one of his attempts.

Elias Håkansson
on 2020

“ I was living in Växjö in 2020, and Daniel and I would train together sometimes. It was up in the air if there would be an Olympics that summer or even in 2021. One day, we were sitting in a restaurant talking about all the uncertainty. It seemed like the only way the Olympics would happen at all was if someone came up with an effective vaccine for Covid right away, but to me that did not seem possible. I knew in the past it took three or four years to develop a vaccine. But Daniel didn't have three or four years. Look how good he was in 2019 and 2020. That was his time to win an Olympic gold, but then Fate stepped in and put a big wall around the time period when he was at his best and said, "Sorry, no Olympics this year."

When I told Daniel it might be years before we had a vaccine, he said, "Well, I guess I'm not going to be Olympic champion then."

That was in April of 2020. ”

WL Marks — Daniel Ståhl

World Leading Marks		Place	
2016:	68.72m	Sollentuna,	SWEDEN
2017:	71.29m NR	Sollentuna,	SWEDEN
2018:	69.72m	Eskilstuna,	SWEDEN
2019:	71.86m NR	Bottnaryd,	SWEDEN
2020:	71.37m	Sollentuna,	SWEDEN
2021:	71.40m	Bottnaryd,	SWEDEN
2022:	71.47m	Uppsala,	SWEDEN

Statistics courtesy of Priit Tänava

These two meets were the ugliest I had seen him throw in years, but a week later in Helsingborg, he reached 70.25m, which made me very happy. To keep his focus, Daniel needed to have fun and there was nothing more fun for him than throwing 70 meters.

Daniel reached 70 meters again at Sollentuna in August and for the rest of the season was consistently around 69 meters. His 71.37m mark from Sollentuna ended up being the best throw in the world for the year, the fifth time in a row he achieved this.

Overall, I was happy with the way we managed 2020. Daniel obviously did not have his best season, but he kept himself together under very difficult circumstances. This would have been his Olympics to win, and the way he handled the disappointment of having the Games postponed was an indication of how much he had matured. Now, we waited to see if he would get his chance at Olympic gold in 2021.

Shaun Pickering
on the 2020 season

" The 2020 season was so strange. We all struggled. Because of Covid, we couldn't go on training camps, and that was especially hard on Daniel. He's always in the public eye in Sweden, so training in a place like Chula Vista is very relaxing for him. Nobody in America knows him really, and there are lots of big people there, so he doesn't stand out so much. He gets to hang out with a small group of people he knows and likes, and he gets to just lift and throw. But there was just no way to manage it in 2020. "

Simon Pettersson
on the Covid Lockdown

" We were on our way to Portugal for a training camp before the Winter Throwing Cup. We had a throwing session on a Monday and were supposed to leave on a Tuesday. I booked my train ticket to Copenhagen to fly to Portugal just after the session, then an hour later Vésteinn called and said we can't go because of the outbreak. We thought it would be a couple weeks, then everything can go back to normal, but that was not the case.

For me, it was not as big of a deal as it was for Daniel. I would have another year to prepare and get better for the Games, but it was tough for Daniel because 2020 was his time. "

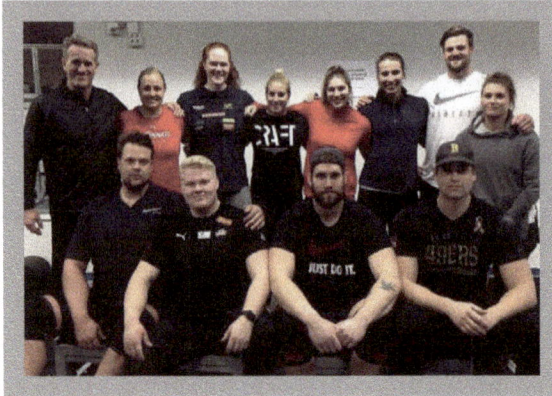

Two training groups in Växjö, Vésteinn with his group and Johanna Vikström with her group. Vésteinn, Frida Åkerström, Daniella Persson, Fanny Roos, Emma Ljungberg, Jennifer Rudberg, Simon Pettersson and Johanna. Daniel, Marcus Thomsen, Viktor Gardenkrans, Jacob Gardenkrans

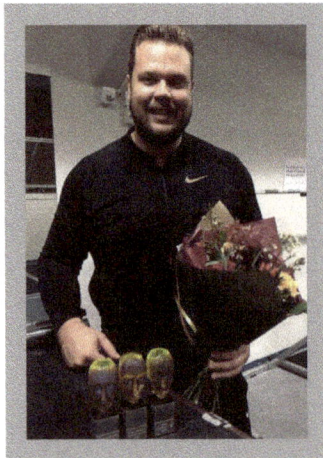

Daniel with three Federation prizes for his 2020 performances

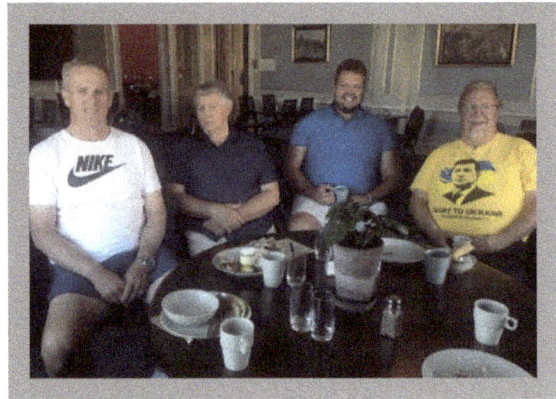

With Jan Ståhl and Jonas Mellblom eating lunch, in Växjö and very often also Tommy Tape is with us

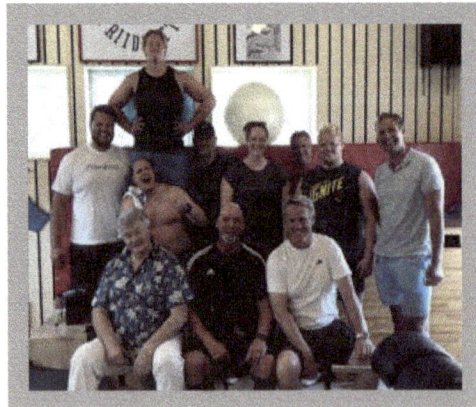

Training at Hässelby IP in Stockholm

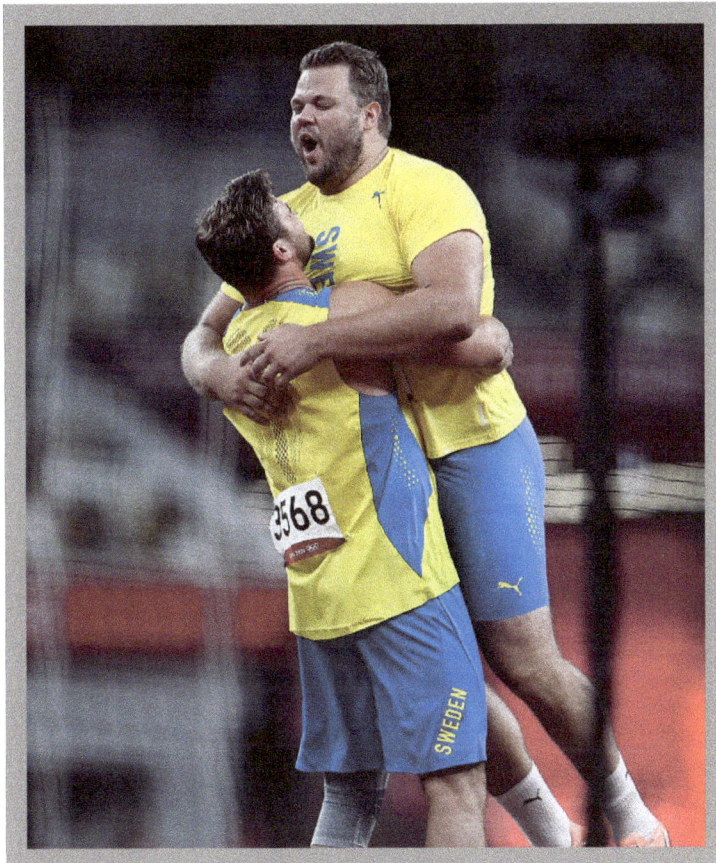

Daniel and Simon celebrate their medals in Tokyo

## 11

2021 — To the Top of the Mountain

As we began training for the 2021 season, Daniel faced big challenges. He had worked hard to become the best discus thrower in the world, but now he would have to deal with the pressure of being a favorite at the Olympic Games. Daniel knew the people of Sweden expected him to take a gold medal in Tokyo and would be disappointed with anything less.

This was understandable based on how well Daniel performed in 2019 and 2020. But, at some point an athlete's skills start to diminish. It happens with everyone, and there is no telling exactly when the decline will begin. There is also no telling when younger athletes might step forward, like when Daniel, Gudžius, and Mason Finley took over the podium at the 2017 Worlds. If Daniel lost a little bit of his edge in 2021 and some other guys made a big jump, it might cost him his chance to win Olympic gold.

This was a lot to think about for a guy who had always struggled with self-doubt, so a big part of my job in 2020-2021 was to keep him focused, keep him on track, and keep his confidence up.

In order to do this, I asked him to stay mostly in Växjö when we began our training in the fall of 2020. Over the years, we always tried to figure out the right balance of how much time Daniel would spend in Växjö and how often he would travel to Stockholm. Earlier in his career, too much time in Växjö would cause him to feel homesick and lose focus. But now, I thought he was ready to stay in town at least 90% of the time, which

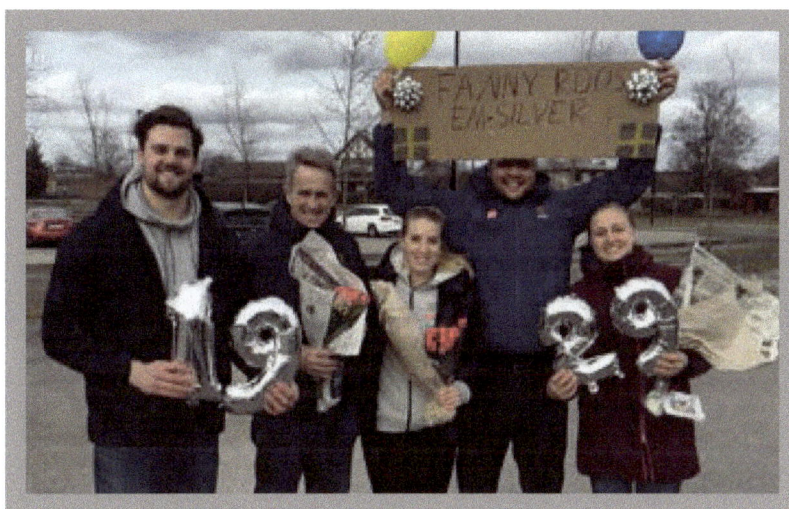

Our year in 2021 started out well with a silver medal by Fanny in the EIC in Torun, Poland

would allow me to give him a maximum amount of attention as he prepared for the Olympics. It would also give me a chance to provide him with daily encouragement and reminders to focus only on what we could control.

Tight focus was still necessary during the winter of 2020-2021 because Covid continued to impact our situation. As I mentioned, we usually went to several training camps in the winter and spring, often to South Africa in January, Portugal in March, and California in April. Daniel is much happier when throwing outdoors in nice weather, so he looks forward to those camps, but we had to cancel all of them due to the pandemic.

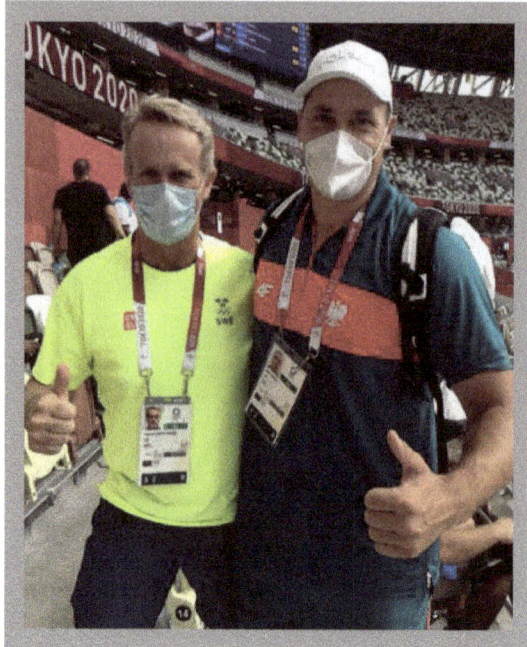

Vésteinn and Gerd meet again as coaches at the 2020 Olympics

Also, there was uncertainty about whether the Olympics would even be held in the summer of 2021. For much of the winter and spring, it seemed possible they might be canceled.

Daniel did a great job dealing with the uncertainty. He trained with energy and focus, and during the winter of 2020-2021 he produced many far throws in our practice hall, including a best of 68.80m, exactly the same as his best training throw in 2019.

There were times when it seemed he was handling the pressure better than I was. There was no escaping the fact that anything less than a gold medal in Tokyo would feel like failure to me as well as to Daniel, and I was determined we would not fail. On many nights I woke up, could not fall back asleep, and instead watched video of some of Daniel's best performances while trying to figure out ways to help him throw even farther.

Going into our annual indoor competition in Växjö on March 7th, I thought Daniel had a chance to break Gerd's unofficial indoor world record of 69.51m, but it was not to be. The atmosphere in the hall was very low key, with Daniel and Simon the only high-level discus throwers in the field and no spectators due to Covid restrictions.

Christoph Harting
on Daniel's Friendship

I can't recall when I met Daniel for the first time, but as far as I remember he's been there ever since. The first time I took note of him actively was at the World Championships in Beijing back in 2015. It was my second major championships, and I was overloaded with nervousness in the qualification as well as in the final. Daniel was around, and he was a pretty funny guy to talk to and to help me unload a bit of excess energy. We had quite a lot of fun, and in the end, he finished fifth and me eighth, if I'm not wrong. I remember that I thought to myself, "I hope we do a couple more meetings and championships together, because I like this guy!"

As time went by, we spent more meetings and time together as I had imagined. But as well as a sporting career is a thing to pass, so is life. The biggest impression comes when you least expect it.

Fast forward to the Kuortane Games in 2021. Life had given us one of its toughest challenges. The virus spread and threw everything all over, including the scheduled Olympic Games.

The year before, a lot of my life broke apart and I found myself in some kind of serious trouble, on and off the field. When depression hit me the hardest and it became clear that I wouldn't make it to the Games, I found myself in preparation for a competition in Finland—Kuortane, a place I'd never heard of and probably won't ever again. The night before the competition, Daniel sent me a message, asking me if I was still awake. It was 10 p.m., but because of the northern hemisphere I would've guessed it was still afternoon. Anyway, we met up half an hour later going into the lake. Yes, bathing in the end of June, in Finland, after 10 p.m., with the sunset as low as it gets at that time of year. Also with us were Simon Pettersson and Kristjan Čeh. And we had quite a chat as we went half a mile into the water until it met our bellies.

Daniel and I fell a bit off, and he asked me how life is going. It broke me—in a good way, I guess. Trying to hold back tears and trying to explain how hard life hit me in the last year and probably would in the upcoming months. He stood there and listened. Listened more than I would've ever expected someone to listen. A guy who grew as a competitor and became a friend over time listened to the depressing life story of another competitor who became a friend of him.

I admire this image and the whole scenery to be honest. Giant human beings (as we are as discus throwers), standing half a mile deep inside of a lake with water at our waist level, talking about the roughest challenges of life trying to help and support each other. But he not only listened, he also gave me some advice and offered me help and support as well.

It was a great moment—at least for me—and a couple of months later, life took a necessary turnaround indeed. With professional help, I managed to manoeuvre out of this darkness. But whenever I feel low, physically or emotionally, I like to remember this evening.

For the record, the competition was won by Daniel with 70.55m, with Kristjan coming second throwing 70.35m. These guys were throwing 70m+ as if it's as easy as pie. 99

Daniel never got totally focused, and he ended up fouling all six of his attempts, four of which went into the cage. We measured the two throws he got out of the cage even though he had fouled them, and they turned out to be 67.96m and 68.28m. This showed his capacity was high and his spirits good.

A few weeks later, at a thrower's meet outdoors in Växjö on May 29th, Daniel had one of the most remarkable days I've ever seen in the discus. The conditions were excellent—maybe 20 degrees Celsius (70 degrees Fahrenheit) with just the right wind. I could tell in warmups that Daniel was feeling something magical when he threw over 72 meters twice. The way he was moving, I thought he might break Jürgen Schult's world record of 74.08m which stood since 1986, so I got on the phone to try to get the doping control people there right away. They had to be present for a new record to be valid.

Unfortunately, Daniel got a little too excited when the competition started and had trouble staying in the ring. One of his fouls was 73.83m, but his best valid mark ended up being 69.11m. Simon won the competition with a huge PB of 69.48m, which started him off on his own magical season.

This began a very busy summer of training, traveling, and competing, during which two main obstacles emerged for Daniel to overcome. The first was Kristjan Čeh.

Kristjan, from Slovenia, threw 68.75m in 2020, when he was only twenty-one years old. He is very tall—2.06m (6'9")—and very smooth in the ring.

In June of 2021, Daniel and Kristjan had an epic battle in Kuortane, Finland. Kristjan hit a huge throw of 70.35m on his third attempt, and Daniel answered with 69.99m. Daniel improved to 70.21m on his next throw but was still in second place. Kristjan broke 70 meters again on his sixth attempt (70.22m) which left Daniel with one final chance to overtake him. On the last throw of the competition, Daniel showed the young upstart that he wasn't ready to give up the throne just yet when he hit 70.55m for the win.

I was proud of how Daniel competed that day. He was definitely tired when he stepped in for his last throw in Kuortane, and he also had a lot of pressure on him not to disappoint his fans in Finland. As I said, his mom grew up there, and the Finns love Daniel. He showed a lot of heart by hitting 70.55m for the win that day, which made me feel even better about his chances in Tokyo.

Another obstacle we had to deal with that summer was the unusual number of competitions scheduled in a short period of time. Traveling and competing can be

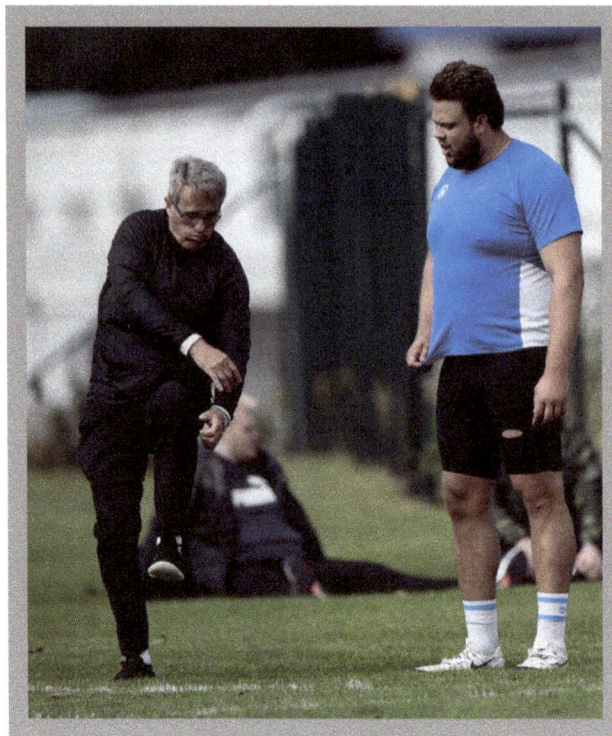

Here I am reminding Daniel to keep his chest forward as long as possible while driving linearly across the ring. This was the technical cue we used going into the Olympic Games.

exhausting, and it is important to have time to recover between meets. But Covid caused some competitions to be rescheduled from early in the 2021 season to a period from late June to early July which was already crowded.

Between June 22nd and July 10th, Daniel and Simon competed seven times while I held my breath, worried they might get injured. Why didn't we simply drop out of a few of those competitions? Well, two of them were Diamond League meetings, and that is where discus throwers can make a little money. One was the Swedish Cup, where athletes represent their clubs, and Daniel and Simon are very loyal to their clubs. As to the others, we gave our word that we would show up, and I always believed that our word should mean something. Luckily, they got through this busy period okay. During one stretch, Daniel threw almost the exact same distance in three consecutive meets (68.65m, 68.65m, and 68.64m) and afterwards I said to him, "Well, we know you'll throw between 68.64m and 68.65m at the Olympics."

Tommy Eriksson
on the training camp in Fukuoka

" It was an easy time in Fukuoka. The Covid protocols did not bother us. If they said to us, "Stand in this queue," we stood in the queue. If we needed to take a Covid test in the morning, we took the test.

Daniel is a social person, so it was easy for him in Fukuoka because he had lots of new friends to hang out with. We played a lot of Yahtzee at first, and I was the champion! The way I was playing, it was like throwing the discus and your first throw goes 72 meters, then your second throw is 71 meters, then 72 once more. After that, I said, "I will never play again," so we switched to card games. But everyone on the Swedish team heard about my Yahtzee skills. The swimmers and football players would come up to me and ask, "Are you Tommy Tape?" That's my nickname. Then they'd look at each other and say, "This is the big champ!" It was like I was a rock star.

It was the best environment for Daniel. Everyone expected him to win the gold medal and playing games and having all those friends around helped him to forget the pressure. "

He finished this hectic period with a huge throw of 71.40m at the Bottnaryd meeting in Sweden, and we were both happy and relieved he had made it through those crazy two weeks without injury. The fact that he finished off this stretch with a world-leading throw was icing on the cake. Next came our trip to Japan for a two-week training camp before the Olympics.

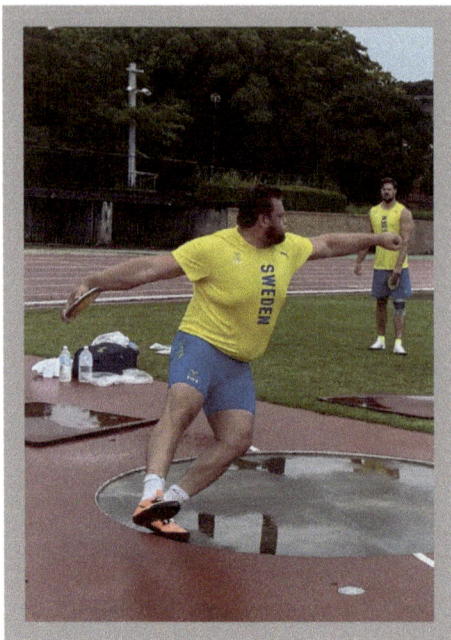

In one of our training sessions in Fukuoka, Japan, before the OG in Tokyo in 2021

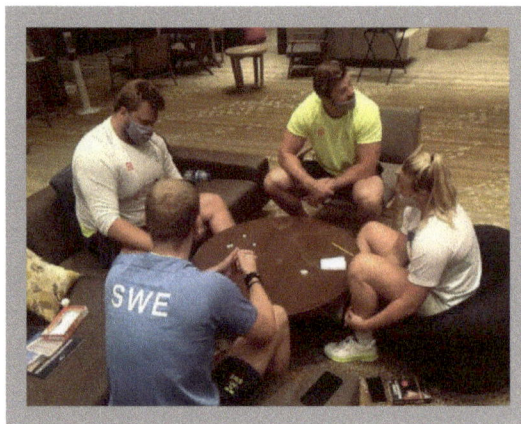

Some time spent relaxing in Fukuoka

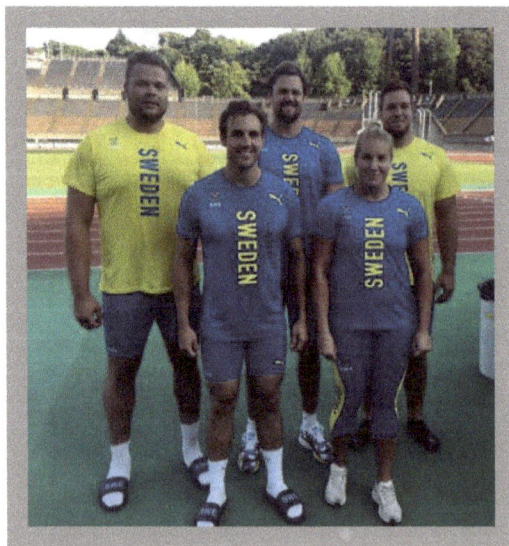

The Swedish throwing team in Fukuoka: Daniel, Kim Amb, Simon, Fanny, Wictor Petersson

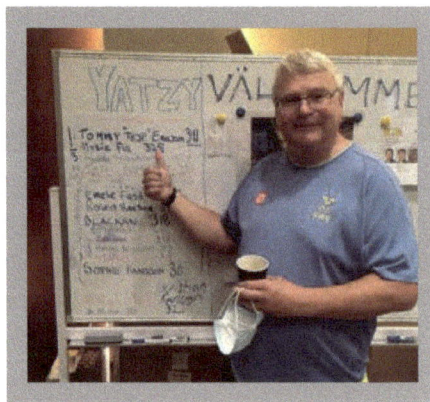

The Yahtzee board of champions, including Tommy "Tape" Eriksson, the happiest man on Earth.

We arrived in Fukuoka, where we would hold our training camp, on July 13th and held our first session the next day.

Our job during this camp was to get acclimated to the time difference and the heat, and to establish a normal rhythm of training so Daniel, Simon, and Fanny would feel comfortable going into the biggest competition of their lives.

This was especially important for Daniel as the pressure was on him to win.

Because of his size, Daniel was more vulnerable to the heat than the others, but we had our physio Tommy Eriksson and our nutritionist Linda Bakkman with us, and they weighed Daniel every morning and evening and tested his urine or saliva each day to make sure he was not getting dehydrated.

We were very lucky to have our full support team with us in Japan, which also included Henrik Wagner, our massage therapist, and Henrik Gustafsson, our mental coach. It was thanks to the Swedish Federation and the Swedish Olympic Committee that we were able to do this.

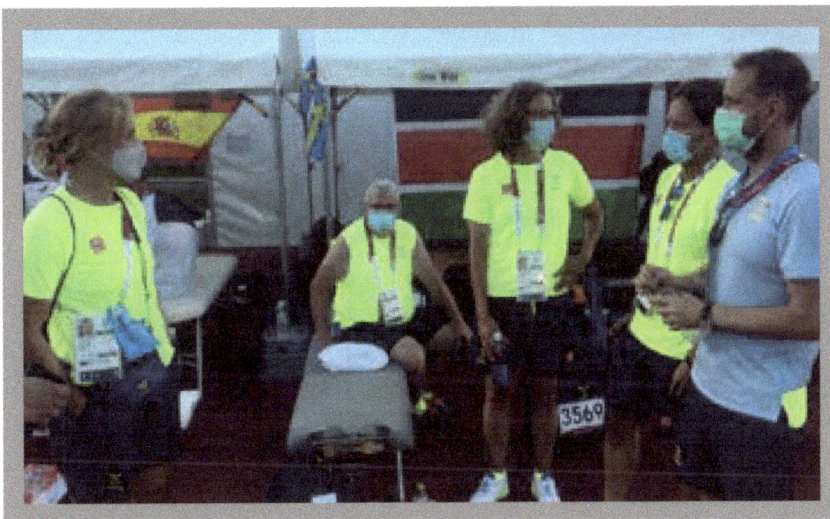

Photo courtesy of Vésteinn Hafsteinsson

On the warmup field with the support team: Hillevi Thor in charge of media, Tommy Tape, Karin Head Coach, Henrik Wagner massage therapist and Henrik Gustafsson mental coach

Simon Pettersson
on the team atmosphere in Fukuoka

" Members of the Swedish team were allowed on three floors of the hotel, and since we were all together it was a good opportunity to get to know the other Swedish athletes better. There was a ping pong table we could use. I played a lot against the soccer girls. And we played a lot of card games. We kept a list displayed of the top ten people in Yahtzee. Daniel played a lot, but our physio, Tommy Eriksson, finished on top with 342 points. He was extremely proud of that.

I shared a room with Daniel, and in one way it was a tense situation for him because of all the pressure to take the gold medal, but the team atmosphere we had in Fukuoka really helped. When you have some other stuff to do, you don't need to think about the seriousness and the expectations. You can relax your mind between training sessions. Daniel is a very social guy, so he needs the stuff that is around the training more than some other people. Sometimes, the stuff around the training is more important than the training because as long as he is happy and enjoying himself, he is going to perform well.

He enjoyed spending time with everyone in Fukuoka, and that was a big key to his success. "

I was confident that with the help of our support team, we would have Daniel ready for the qualification round on July 30th, and all went as planned. He threw and lifted well during our camp in Fukuoka, and after a few days felt comfortable with the heat and the time change.

Looking back, I also think the Covid situation might have helped Daniel deal with the pressure of being the gold medal favorite. Swedish athletes from all sports were together at the training camp in Fukuoka, and because our movements were restricted, we spent most of our free time in a large communal room playing ping pong and video games and Yahtzee.

It was the best environment for Daniel. Playing games and having all those friends around helped him to forget the pressure.

We flew into Tokyo two days before the discus qualification, and Daniel seemed calmer than he had been in Doha two years before.

It helped that life in the Olympic Village felt nearly the same as at any other Olympic Games. We had to continue following Covid protocols—daily testing, masking, wearing

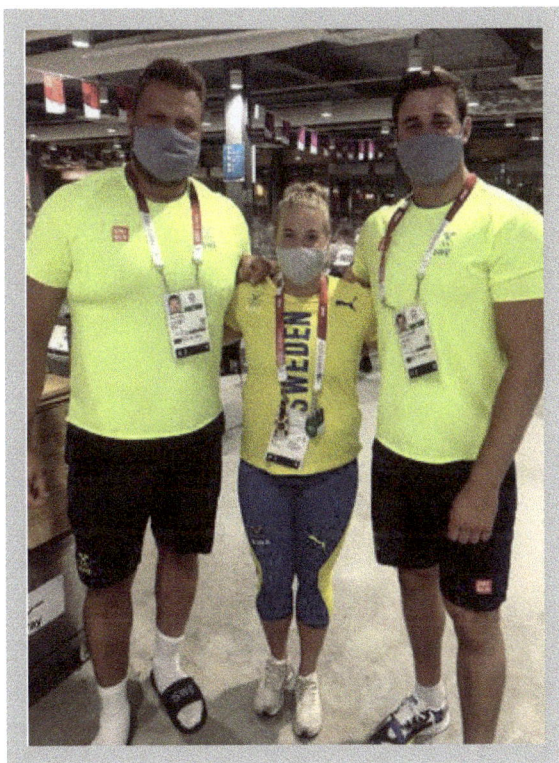

In the cafeteria in the Olympic Village

Shaun Pickering
on the Tokyo Olympics

> " I sat with Vésteinn during the final in Tokyo. He is pretty intense at those moments, and he forgets about himself, so years ago I promised his wife Anna that I would look after him as best I could. I'm famous for always having my backpack with me, and when I know I'm going to sit with Vésteinn, I'll keep drinks and snacks in there for him.
>
> When we sat down for the final in Tokyo, the first thing I did was hand him a drink and a sandwich. "

gloves in the cafeteria—but we could move around the Village freely, and everyone ate in a huge dining hall that was two levels and could hold something like 10,000 people. It was fun seeing athletes from all over the world there. I got a picture with the weightlifter Lasha Talakhadze, who won the gold in Rio and again in Tokyo in the super-heavyweight category. He looks a lot stronger than me in the photo, but that is just the camera angle.

As I described earlier, Daniel loves socializing, so having the opportunity to mix with other athletes in the Olympic Village was good for him.

The dormitory in the Olympic Village was made up of apartments with three or four bedrooms and a living room in each. My roommate was Björn Amb, father of the javelin thrower Kim Amb, who was Swedish champion nine times. Kim ended up performing well in Tokyo, throwing a season's best of 82.40m in qualification and finishing eleventh in the final.

The qualification round for men's discus was on the morning of July 30th. I rode the bus to the stadium with Simon and Daniel, and then took a seat with a clear view of the discus cage. Because of Covid, only athletes, journalists, and team officials were allowed inside, so the stands were almost empty. A lot of people asked me later if the strange conditions at these Olympics bothered us, but by that point in the pandemic, strange had become normal and we barely even noticed the lack of spectators.

I sat alone in the stands, but my friend Shaun Pickering was close by as were Karin Torneklint and a few others from the Swedish squad. Karen was the team captain for Sweden and did everything she could to help Daniel succeed. It was because of Karin that we were able to have our full support team of Tommy, Linda, and both Henriks with us in Fukuoka and Tokyo.

It gave Daniel extra confidence to have them there, which was good because before the qualification round began, he launched both of his warmup throws into the cage!

When he came over to speak with me before his first competition attempt, I just said, "Move one foot to the left in the circle when you set up and get those throws out of the cage."

He did and tossed a nice, easy 66.12m on his first attempt. The automatic qualifying mark was 66.00m, so after one throw Daniel's job was done and he left to take the bus back to the Village.

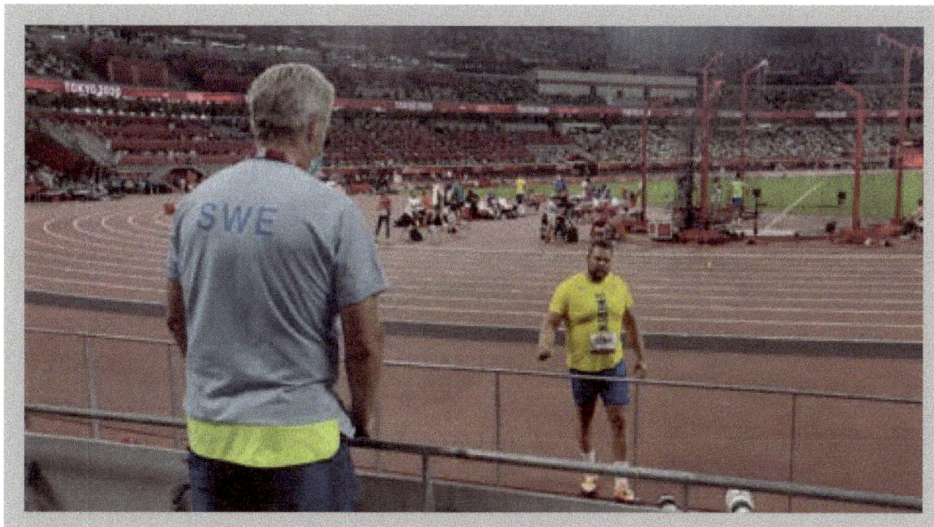

The coach and the athlete in action in Tokyo OG 2021

Photo courtesy of Shaun Pickering

Simon was in the second group for qualification, and the process was not as easy for him. His first throw was 60.62, and his second was only 59.47m.

Shaun and Karin were freaking out a little bit, but I stayed calm. Simon's worst result in any meet during the 2021 season was 63.03m. If he could just equal that on his third throw in qualification, he would likely advance. For sure, being down to one last throw to qualify can be an unnerving experience. At a moment like that, it is easy to let fear of failure take over and paralyze you. But Simon never thinks about failing during big competitions. He always believes his next throw will be a big one. He does not defeat himself like some others do.

Simon showed this mental toughness once again by throwing 64.18m on his third attempt, which placed him seventh and put him in the final with room to spare.

The final was scheduled for the evening on July 31st. My athletes always do a brief morning workout on the day of a competition in order to get loose and wake up their nervous system. Daniel likes to take a walk for his "wakeup call," and he did this on his own in the Olympic Village. I took Simon out for a few drills and easy throws, and when we returned, I sat with him and Daniel for a brief talk.

"Remember," I told them. "Tonight, we stay with our plan. We will not do anything special or unusual. We have our cues. We practiced them many times in Fukuoka. If you come to me for advice between throws, I will tell you to stick to your cue."

When I say "cue" I mean a simple technical point that I give each of my athletes to focus on during a competition. The cue is meant to help them switch to autopilot and let their feel and instincts take over when they step into the ring.

I described earlier how challenging it can be for a thrower to keep their mind calm during a qualification round. It is the same at an Olympic final, which is always the biggest moment in a thrower's career, much bigger even than a World Championships, though the level of competition is the same. At an Olympics, it feels like the entire world is watching, and this can make it difficult to relax and focus on the task at hand.

This is where our cues come in.

By focusing on one small bit of technique, we reduce the most stressful night of a thrower's career to the repetition of a simple task which they have rehearsed many times. Counting warmup throws, they repeat the task eight or nine times during competition. How hard can that be?

The cue we decided on for Daniel in Tokyo was to drive linearly across the ring while keeping his chest facing forward as long as possible. For Simon it was to start the throw early with his left side so he would get a long path out of the back.

After meeting with the guys, I spent the day walking around and drinking coffee, feeling the heat in my palms and feeling like I was going to throw up—business as usual for me at a major championships.

Finally, the hours passed, and it was time to take the bus to the stadium. When we arrived, I once again took a seat by myself, but with Shaun sitting one row behind over my left shoulder, and Tommy Eriksson one row behind over my right shoulder.

During a championship final, I like to be in my own bubble, but it also feels good to have people I trust close by. I worked with Tommy for many years. He was a huge part of the team we assembled around Daniel. And Shaun was an old friend whose advice I relied on many times, so it gave me comfort to have him and Tommy there. And since I sat near Shaun at every major championships since 2007, he knew I was usually too nervous to think about eating, so he always thought ahead to put sandwiches and bottles of water in his bag for me. That's the kind of guy he was, always taking care of everyone else.

So, as the discus warmups began, I was sitting in the stands alone but not alone, and feeling at peace with how the night would go. It is a strange thing with me, but I often get a feeling before a competition of how things will turn out. Sometimes I know we are going to do well, and sometimes I know we are not. In 2009, Gerd was defending World and Olympic champion. Going into the World Championships in Berlin, he was undefeated on the season and had thrown at least 69 meters in eight different competitions. But, for some reason, I got a bad feeling the day of the final. It seemed like there was something that should be there but was not there. That night, he threw 66.88m and finished third while Robert Harting took the gold and ran around tearing his shirt to pieces. That was the changing of the guard in the men's discus, as Robert went on to win two more World titles and an Olympic gold medal.

I have had a bad feeling before other competitions over the years, and it makes the hours go by very slowly as you sit around waiting for the disaster and knowing you cannot control it.

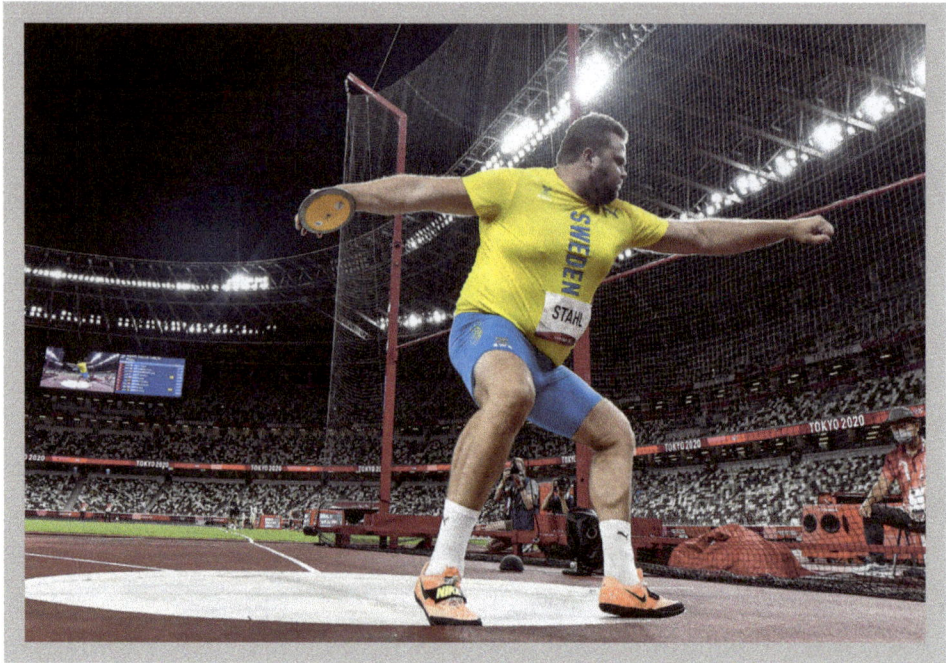

Daniel about to launch

But on the day of the discus final in Tokyo, I did not feel a disaster coming. As I said, I felt excited and nervous all day like I always do before a big competition, but my main goal in Tokyo was for Daniel to win the gold medal, and I felt sure he would. Why was I so sure about Daniel in 2021 but not about Gerd in 2009 when both were in great shape and had dominated all season? I have no good explanation.

The air in the stadium that night was like a sauna—humid and no breeze whatsoever. It reminded me of my college days in Alabama.

I sat there sweating quietly as Daniel and Simon took their warmup throws. If you have prepared properly, there is not much coaching to do during a competition, so I would just watch and only talk to my athletes if they came to me. Daniel and Simon both looked relaxed and smooth on their warmups, so there was not much to say anyway.

When the competition finally began, none of the main contenders was able to hit a big throw in the first round. Lukas Weißhaidinger, who took the bronze medal at the 2018 Europeans and the 2019 Worlds, was first up of the twelve finalists, and he only did 62.32m.

Karin Torneklint
on the Tokyo Olympics

" It was, of course, a very strange situation in Tokyo, but we were used to dealing with Covid by then. By the time we got to the Olympics, we had no expectations of competing in front of a large crowd, and we didn't care. We just wanted to compete.

As the athletes arrived at our training camp in Fukuoka, we had to always keep the new arrivals separate from those who had been there for a few days in case they accidentally brought Covid with them. The new ones could not share a car with the others or sit with them during a meal.

The athletes had more freedom to mix with others once they got to the Olympic Village in Tokyo. I was very nervous one day when the pole vaulter Sam Kendricks of the United States tested positive. Mondo Duplantis was supposed to have coffee with him that day in the Village, but fortunately they changed plans, and he was not exposed.

It was a lot of stress for everyone, but we tried to do our best, stay calm, and have a good time.

The day of the discus final, I was sitting in the arena a little bit far away from Vésteinn because I didn't want to disturb him while he was coaching. After three rounds, Daniel was winning and Simon was in third, but then on his fifth throw Kristjan Čeh passed Simon, and my phone immediately started going crazy. People from Sweden who were watching on television were calling me to tell me Čeh had fouled on that throw. I got about fifty calls telling me, "You must protest!" They kept sending pictures and films from the broadcast for me to show to the officials.

I ran to the Technical Information Center or "TIC" to file a protest and found myself screaming at the Japanese officials. "You've got to take that throw away! It is not correct!"

They calmly told me that I must fill out a certain paper. The Japanese, as you may know, are very formal. I could not see the competition from inside the TIC, so I kept checking my phone while I filled out the form. Finally, I called our media person, Hillevi Thor.

"What is happening in the competition? I'm sitting here trying to get them to fix this wrong decision!"

"Oh," she said. "It's no problem anymore. Simon threw farther. He is in second place now!"

I immediately told the Japanese, "I don't care about this anymore," and tried to leave to go back to the seats, but they said once you start the process you must finish it.

I said, "No! I must go celebrate!" and they finally let me go after I promised to come back and finish filling out the form.

Simon's first throw was 61.39m, but it was normal for him to open not so well, so I wasn't worried.

Daniel began with a throw that went straight up in the air and landed at 63.72m. He came over to talk afterwards, and I just told him to stick to his cue.

Kristjan's first attempt was over 65 meters, but he fouled it by stepping on top of the ring on his finish.

Andrius Gudžius was the last thrower in the order, and he started well with 64.05m, but when the first round ended Matty Denny from Australia was in the lead with 65.76m. This was close to his season's best of 66.15m, which is impressive for a thrower competing in his first Olympics. As I described earlier, Gerd and Daniel both struggled in their first Games, but some athletes have a knack for competing on the big stage even when they are young, and Denny is one of them.

Lukas took over the lead at the beginning of round two with a throw of 66.65m. Then another young guy, Sam Mattis from the United States, hit a season's best of 63.88m.

Denny had another nice throw (65.53m) on his second attempt, and next up after him was Simon.

When Simon stepped into the ring, Lukas (66.65m) was in first, Denny (65.76m) in second, and Gudžius (64.05m) in third.

As I said earlier, Simon is a guy who loves the spotlight, and he showed it by throwing 66.58m to take over second place!

That distance made it very likely he would finish no worse than fifth, which was my goal for him coming into Tokyo. When he came over to the railing, I told him the pressure was off, our job was done, and he could be happy. But in his mind, he was not done. "There's more where that came from!" he assured me, and he could hardly wait to get back in the cage for his third throw.

A couple of minutes later, Daniel walked in to take his second attempt. Many years had passed since the first time I traveled to Stockholm to watch him throw. His life was simple then. All he wanted to do was play hockey, hang out with his friends, go hunting and fishing with his dad, lift heavy weights in his local gym and throw a little discus for his club. Then I showed up and got him to dream about winning an Olympic gold medal. Together, we went on a long journey to make that dream happen, but there were moments along the way when it must have seemed more like a nightmare for Daniel, like early on, when he had to spend so much time away from Stockholm, the place where he was happy, or later when he made the big throw at Irvine and the spotlight was put on him. As big and strong as Daniel is, carrying the weight of his country's expectations almost broke him, and there were times he wanted nothing more than to go back to living a simple, anonymous life in Stockholm. But he always summoned the courage to endure, and together we kept chasing the dream. The chase led us finally to this big, humid, empty stadium in Tokyo, and as Daniel entered the ring for his second throw, every mask-covered face turned to watch him. In the Village, Swedish athletes from all the various sports started yelling at their computer screens. Millions of people in Sweden did the same. But the stadium was quiet as Daniel took his windup, sprinted through the ring and launched his discus into the heavy air.

It came down at 68.90m, the fourth longest throw in Olympic history. And now, Daniel was in first place.

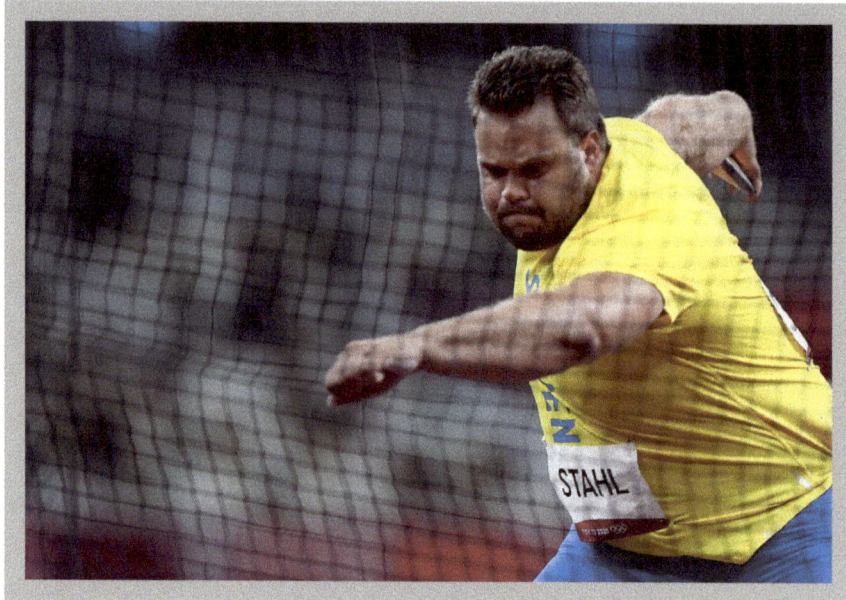

Daniel carried the expectations of his entire country into the Olympic Games
and came through as a champion.

That throw did not guarantee Daniel the gold medal, but it made things very hard
on the guys chasing him. Obviously, Kristjan had the capacity to throw far. I heard later
that his foul in the first round was 67 meters, and he had thrown 70.35m at Kuortane
in June. But at that point in his career, Kristjan had only thrown 68 meters or better
four times, so it did not seem likely that he would do it again under pressure in a big
stadium on a humid night. In fact, his second-round throw of 62.95m left him vulnerable
to being knocked out of the top eight, which would mean his night would be over after
three throws.

Gudžius was the 2017 World Champion, and had thrown 68 or better many times,
but only once in 2021. Simon threw 69.48m in June with great conditions in Växjö,
but that was the only time he had ever been over 68 meters. Matty Denny's PB coming
into the Olympics was 66.15m. Weißhaidinger was the guy who scared me the most.
He had a PB of 69.04m and an unusual technique where he looked extremely fast but
out of control. Whenever we competed against him, I always worried that everything

would fall into place, and he would produce a huge throw. On this night in Tokyo, he had four more chances to do it.

After the 68.90m, Daniel was leading with Weißhaidinger second at 66.65m and Simon third with his 66.58m.

When Daniel came over to talk, I told him that the 68.90m had him in a good spot so maybe it was time to push a little harder on the gas pedal and see what would happen. I was hoping he might be able to break the Olympic record of 69.89m that Virgilijus Alekna set in 2004.

Lukas improved to 67.07m to begin the third round, and Denny threw a little better too, but his 65.94m did not get him into the top three. Simon released his third throw a little early, and it landed out of bounds to the right. Daniel did go harder on his third attempt, but his timing was off, and the disc went almost straight up in the air. It shows how much power he put behind the throw that it still traveled 65.16m.

Kristjan threw poorly on his third attempt, then had to stand and watch as Chad Wright of Jamaica came very close to knocking him out of the competition. Lucky for him,

Hans Üürike
on a conversation with Piotr Malachowki

> I remember a conversation I had with Piotr Malachowski at a meeting in Turku earlier in the 2021 season. Piotr came up to me and said, "Hans, you know I am an experienced discus thrower, and I am telling you Daniel will win no problem. But the dark horse for Tokyo is Simon."
>
> After the Games, I wrote to Piotr and asked, "How in the hell did you know?"
>
> He just said, "Hey, I am an experienced discus thrower."

Wright's throw was 62.56m. Kristjan's best was 62.95m, so he stayed in eighth place and received three more attempts.

The group was re-ordered after the first three rounds, and Kristjan led off the fourth round with a big improvement of 66.05m. Gudžius (64.11m) continued to struggle, and Matty Denny continued his remarkably consistent night with a throw of 65.00m. Simon was a little off on his release, but still hit 66.24m. Lukas threw 66.86m, and Daniel 66.10m, so the top three remained the same: Daniel, Lukas, then Simon.

Drama came at the beginning of round five when Kristjan threw 66.62m to jump Simon. As soon as that throw was posted, though, Karin Torneklint started getting messages from people in Sweden who saw on the slow-motion replay that Kristjan had probably fouled. She texted to give me a heads up and immediately went to file a protest, but it did not matter because when Simon's next turn came, he smashed a throw of 67.39m to move all the way up to second place! Later, he told me getting passed by Kristjan had fired him up, another sign of what a great competitor Simon is.

Denny improved to 66.06m in the fifth round, but Lukas fouled his throw and Daniel hit 67.03m, so with one round remaining, the top three were now Daniel, Simon, then Lukas.

As the sixth and final round began, I could not bear to watch anymore and instead went out to the concourse to pace. Some journalists sitting near me were puzzled by this, but by then the tension was just too much and I had to get away. So, I did not see Kristjan make his best throw of the night (66.37m) or Gudžius finish with a foul, or Matty Denny throw a PB of 67.02m, just a few centimeters short of taking the bronze medal from Lukas. Before the sixth round they re-made the order so the leaders would come at the end and have a chance to respond if someone jumped them. Because of this, Lukas was the last guy who had a chance to knock my guys out of first and second. When it came up on my phone that he fouled his final throw, I could no longer control my emotions and I came running down the aisle screaming. Dane Miller, the coach of Sam Mattis, jumped up and gave me a hug, and so did Tommy and probably others too, but I was so excited I can't remember exactly.

Simon threw 65.39m to finish his incredible night, and then Daniel entered the ring as the new Olympic champion.

He was full of emotion and only threw 64.58m on his final attempt, but it didn't matter. Someone tossed the guys Swedish flags, and as I watched them celebrate, I felt very odd. I was the happiest coach in history, and I also knew this moment could never be topped. It was a combination of happiness and emptiness. But that is the life of a coach!

I was immensely proud of both those guys, especially Daniel after everything he'd overcome to make it to the top of the Olympic podium.

After he won, Daniel held up the Swedish flag and started yelling, "I am a Swedish Viking!"

He was also an Olympic champion and hero to the Swedish people, amazing to consider when you think about what he went through.

Later, some time after that night in Tokyo, I looked over at Daniel one day during a training session and saw he was getting emotional. I asked him what was the matter, and

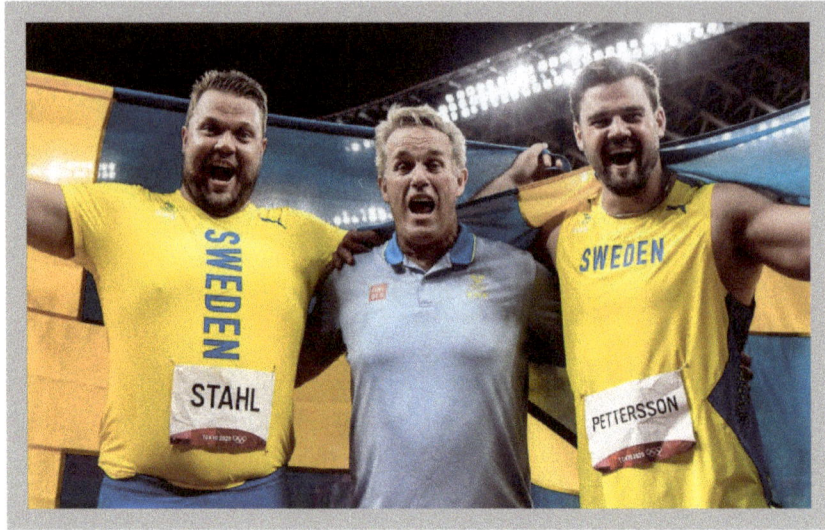

Crazy Times

he said, "I was just thinking about everything we have done. It makes me so happy when I think about where I could be right now if things had gone a different way."

I think about that often as well, and I have to say the thing I am happiest about when I look back on my career is the way the big, crazy, uncontrollable kid I first met at a throwing cage in Stockholm in 2010 grew to be a good man who is kind and thoughtful and has a bright future ahead of him after he is done throwing, a future that I hope will include becoming a husband and father, because he is ready to be great at both those roles.

Simon Pettersson
on that Incredible Night in Tokyo

66 It had been a career goal of mine to take a medal at a major championship and celebrate with the Swedish flag, and when the competition was over, there I was with Daniel, each of us holding a flag while people took pictures. Then Daniel sprinted off, and I started following him, but after about sixty meters he started gasping, so we decided to end our victory lap there.

It took some time to finish up at the stadium, and it was around 1:30 a.m. when we got back to the village. The whole handball team and some others were standing outside the hotel cheering and singing. It was very special, a very nice feeling–a team feeling. I felt it already in the pre-camp. Everyone was so kind to each other and created an atmosphere where everyone was included, everyone was part of the group. Then, when all those people were standing there waiting for us it showed that everyone was part of the same team.

The Prime Minister called us, which was an unreal feeling after you have heard his voice on television for many years. He told us how he and his wife had watched the discus competition together.

Later, when we got home, we had all kinds of people congratulating us. One of the reasons I am throwing the discus is to make something good in this world, and it seemed like maybe we had done that. 99

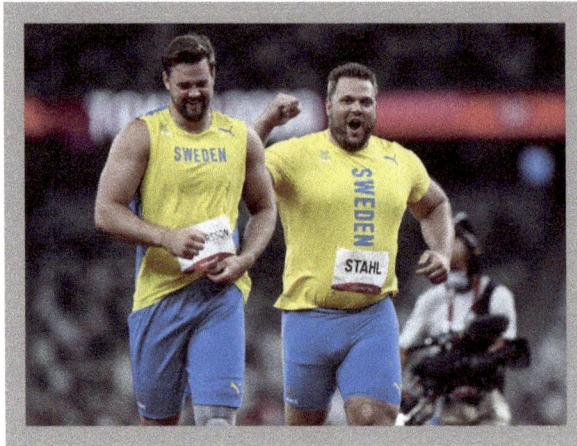

Simon and Daniel
are overjoyed at their
Olympic success

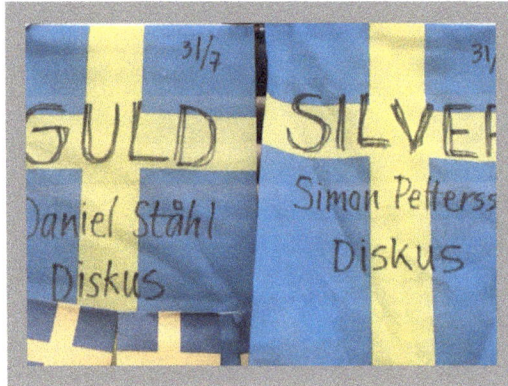

Recognition at the
Swedish team camp

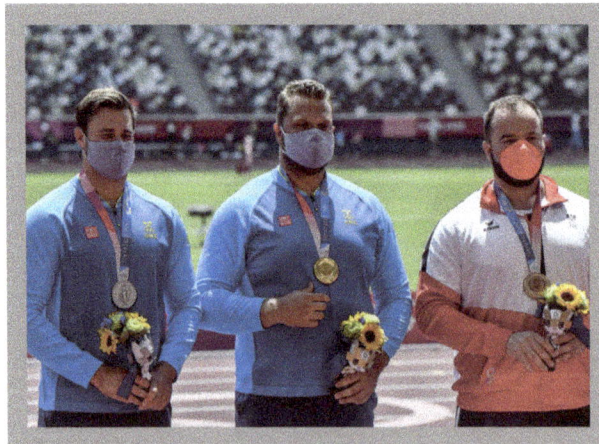

OG medalists
Simon, Daniel and
Lukas Weißhaidinger

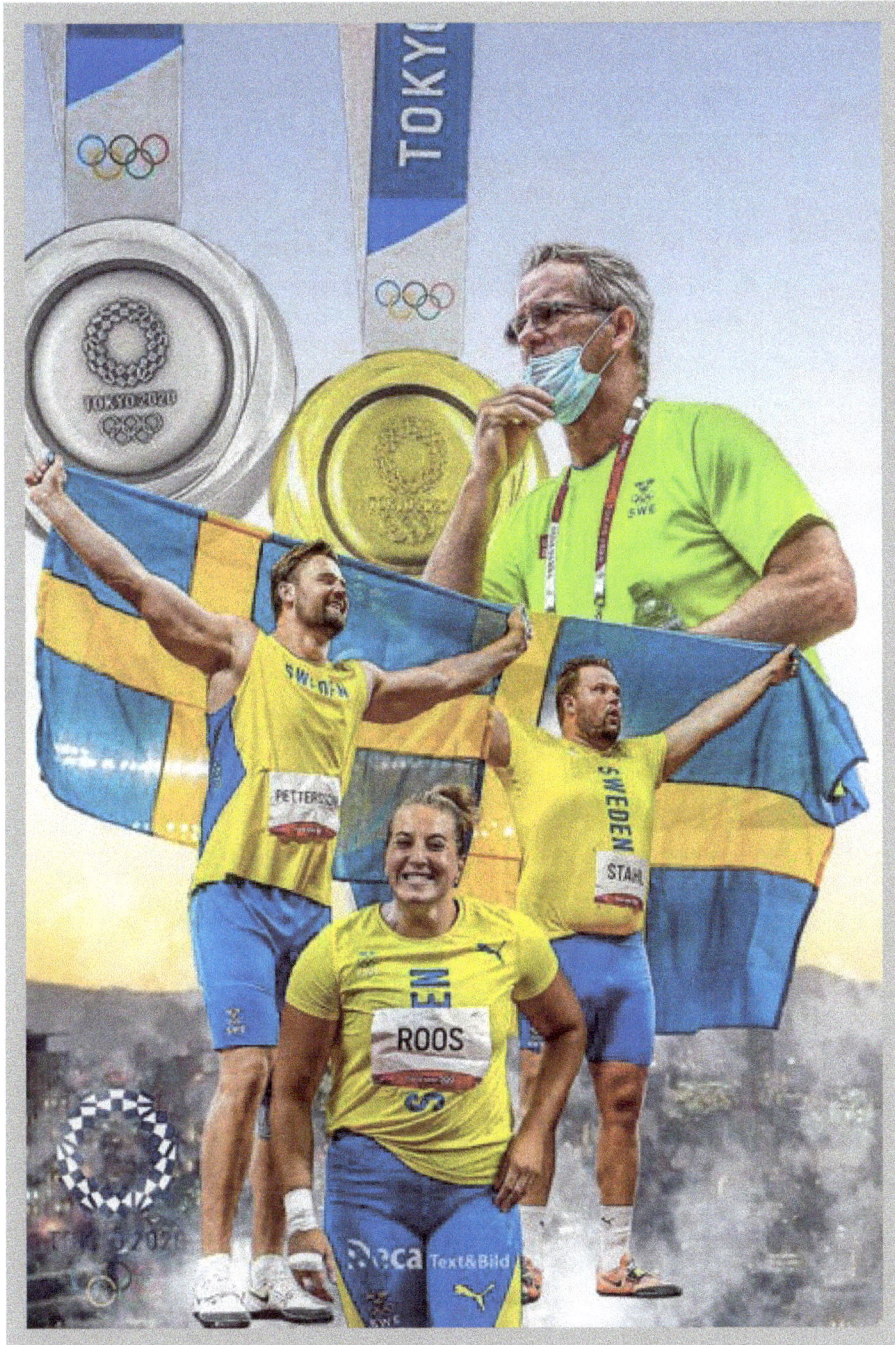

Commemorative Olympic poster designed by Daniel's good friend, Arwid Koskinen

Hans Üürike
on the Tokyo Olympics

"Because of Covid, managers like me were not allowed to go to Tokyo, so I watched the highlight of my career on TV with my wife. We both wore Swedish national shirts. It was like a dream the way everything worked out. Daniel threw his season average and won, and Simon exceeded all expectations by taking the silver medal.

I screamed like crazy here on my couch in Tallinn. My wife recorded my celebration, and I sent it to Daniel. His response was, "Hans, you are a funny manager.""

Kajsa Bergqvist
on watching the Olympic final

"I watched the Olympics on television. My wife and I were at our country house, and the same night as the discus final we were supposed to attend a meeting with the people in our village to discuss road repairs or something. I tried to explain to the chairman of the village that it was absolutely impossible that I could be at this meeting, and he was like, "It's very important! I sent out the notice two months ago!" He was definitely not a sports fan.

The whole time, I was standing up and screaming and sometimes hiding behind a pillow. My wife kept telling me to calm down, but I was like, "You don't understand what is happening!"

When it was over, I ran out into the garden screaming. It is amazing how sport can trigger such emotions."

Fanny Roos
on the Tokyo Olympics

" Our pre-Olympic training camp in Fukuoka was the first one we went to in a long time because of Covid, and it was a really fun camp. Athletes from all the different Swedish teams were there, handball and football and all the other sports. Our training went well, and there was also a room for playing games. We played Yahtzee with all the different athletes, and it was really nice to meet people and have fun and not think so much about Covid. We got tested every day, and we did what we were told to do, but basically, we just trained and played games and had fun.

I watched the men's discus final on television from the Olympic Village because I had my shot put final the next morning.

I watched on a computer with some girls from the swimming team and one weightlifter. It was amazing just to see two people from Sweden take gold and silver, and even more amazing to see Daniel and Simon take gold and silver! I got goosebumps and felt so inspired.

During the last training session in Fukuoka, just two days before the Olympics, I injured my knee and could barely walk. But Tommy Eriksson taped me before I competed, and watching the discus final had me so inspired that I didn't even think about my injury, and I ended up finishing seventh, which made me very happy.

That was an important moment in my career, but seeing Daniel and Simon win the gold and silver medals is my all-time favorite sports memory. "

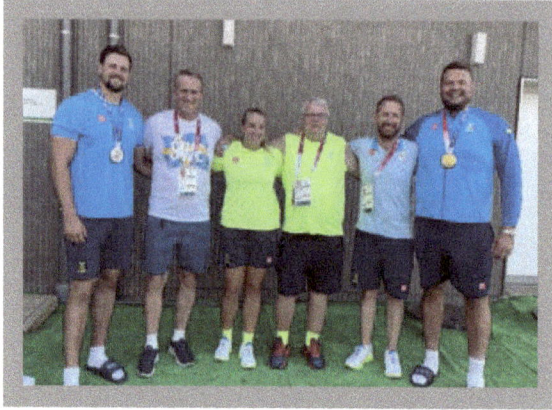

The gang with Tommy Tape the physio and our great mental coach, Henrik Gustafsson

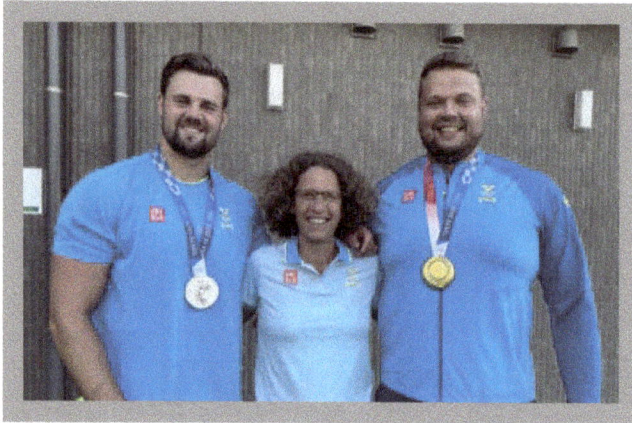

Happy T&F Head Coach Karin Torneklint

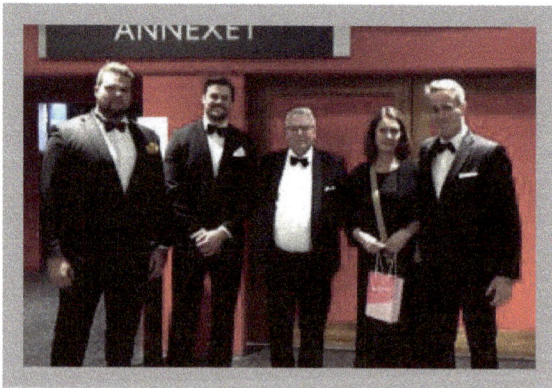

In 2021 when we went to Idrottsgalan, the annual prize ceremony for Swedish sports. Daniel and Simon with the man, Tommy Tape. My wife Anna usually joins me at these festivals.

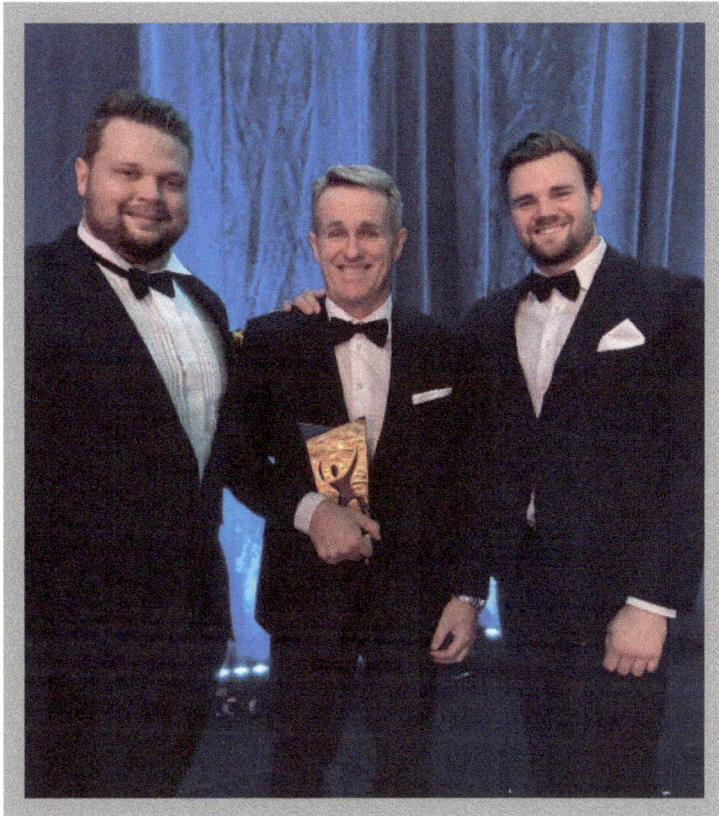

Vésteinn was named 2021 Swedish Coach of the Year

12

2022 — An Unexpected Turn

Things do not always go as they did in Tokyo.

I had four athletes qualify for the 2012 Olympic Games. Kim Christensen, the Danish national shot-put champion, came into London with a PB of 20.06m. He threw 19.13m in qualification and finished 27th. Brett Morse, the British discus thrower, had a PB of 66.06m. He threw 58.18m and finished 35th.

Märt Israel of Estonia hurt himself during our final training session. He was straining to get off a big throw to have confirmation that he would do well in the competition, and he pulled a groin muscle. I should have ended that training session earlier, but I didn't. Märt threw 60.34m in qualification and finished 25th. His PB at the time was 66.98m.

My last thrower to compete in London was Gerd. He was in the second group for qualification, and he opened with a throw into the cage. His second attempt was 59.72m. Keep in mind, Gerd's PB was 73.38.

During the competition, I was sitting in the stands with Raul Rebane. After Gerd's second attempt, I took a trip to the washroom to calm my nerves. And I will never forget standing alone in the bathroom at the London Olympics and thinking, "Ok, Gerd will take his third throw, then he will be out, and all of my guys will have screwed up and my career will be over."

I put on a brave face when I returned to the stands, and assured Raul that Gerd would qualify on his third throw. "He always does," I reminded him. "He has not failed in a qualification round since 2002. But it usually takes him three throws."

"How can you be so cool?" he asked.

"I don't know," I replied. "I guess I just think the sun will always come up tomorrow."

Luckily, Gerd threw 66.39m on his third attempt in qualifying and then hit a season's best 68.03m in the final to take the bronze medal. So, the sun did come up, and my career continued.

Not that this business of coaching got any easier. I have sometimes succumbed to the pressure of expectations myself, and over the years I have come dangerously close to damaging my health. During the 2016 season, I was hospitalized twice with panic attacks.

This is the backside of success. You get caught up in it and then you can never relax, never go to a family party and forget about your job for a couple of hours.

As the 2022 season approached, I started obsessing over how we could improve on what we had accomplished in 2021. I knew at some point Daniel's skills might start to diminish, but I thought if I managed his training correctly, we could delay any decline for another year or two. And with Marcus, Simon and Fanny just entering their prime, I had reason to believe they might take another big step forward. With the World and European Championships coming up in the summer of 2022, I was excited at the possibility of contending for more medals.

But what I did not perceive was how much of a toll the last two years had taken emotionally on my athletes and on me. We had maintained our focus through all the upheavals caused by the pandemic. We had fought our way to the top of the mountain. But it took every ounce of our energy to do it.

After the Tokyo Games, I was overwhelmed with messages of congratulation from former colleagues, mentors, and opponents from all over the world. Mac Wilkins contacted

Tommy Eriksson
on 2022 and beyond

“ Daniel was tired in 2022. That is normal. After you have done a super result in one season, then comes the backlash the next season. It becomes hard to focus one hundred percent because you are not so hungry as you were before you got the result. And the pressure is still there. You throw 67 meters, and everyone says, "He only threw 67 meters," even though that is a pretty good mark. Also, the younger guys coming up only think one thing: "We are going to beat Daniel."

He also found out he could earn a little money because he was the Olympic champion, but then everyone wants something from you, which is distracting.

But I think he will be ok now. He is happy and more balanced in his life than he has ever been. He was disappointed when Vésteinn stepped down, but Daniel is clever in the head, and he understood that Vésteinn wanted to go home to Iceland and that it was time to congratulate him and move forward.

I tell Daniel, "You are strong enough to throw far, you just have to be smart." When he was younger, he could maybe take sixty throws in a session. Now, it is better to take twenty perfect throws and leave it at that. If he does, I think he could still break the world record.

Daniel is looking forward to the 2024 Olympics, and I tell him, after that take it one year at a time. As long as it is fun and you think you can do good things, keep going, maybe all the way to Los Angeles in 2028. After that, we take a one week vacation in Hawaii and then we say goodbye.

I have so appreciated working with him. I call Daniel my little brother, partly because I love him so much, and also because it makes me feel not so old. ”

me, and so did a former discus thrower from Paraguay who Mac coached when I was a young thrower training in California. I had not spoken to the man in thirty years. I heard from my dear friend and former training partner Nick Sweeney, whose suggestion about altering Gerd Kanter's windup many years ago helped make Gerd a 70-meter thrower. Joe Kovacs and Ryan Crouser congratulated me when I saw them after their shotput qualification in Tokyo. Joe knew Daniel and Simon from their early days when I first took them to training camps at Chula Vista. Gerd texted to say he would now call me "Doctor Discus." A woman from my childhood in Iceland who sent me a love letter when I was fourteen years old contacted me. The King of Sweden sent us all a message of congratulations. People in Sweden also messaged my wife, congratulating her on being married to me!

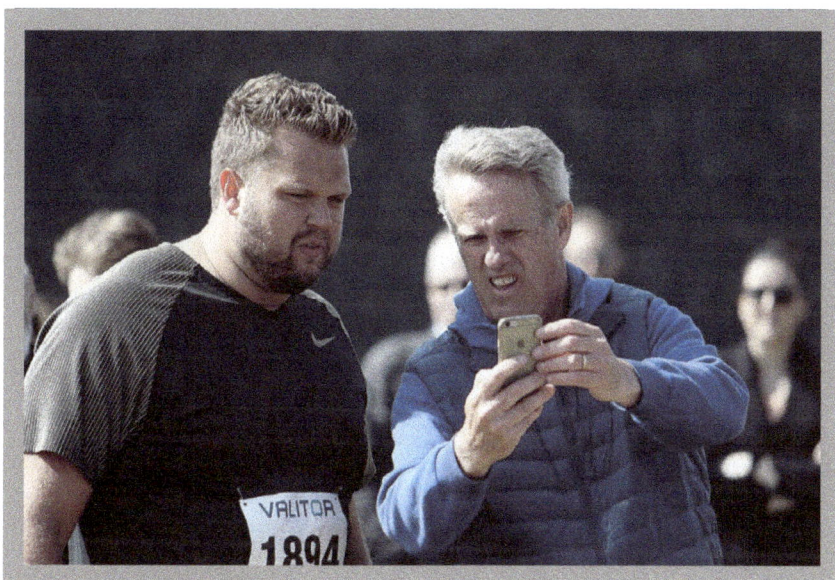

Daniel and I working our way through a difficult 2022 season.

Not long after the Games, the Crown Prince and Princess of Sweden came on an official visit to Växjö. They stopped at different businesses and schools and expressed a special wish to meet up with us. Daniel, Fanny, and I met them at our training hall, and we had a chat about throwing and showed them how we do it. They both tried to

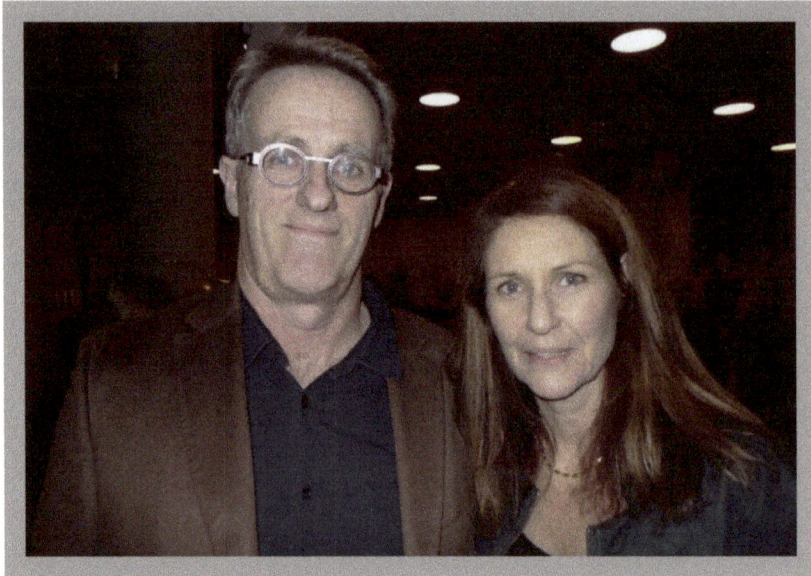

Photo courtesy of Vésteinn Hafsteinsson

Anna supported me through my whole career. In 2022, she told me it was time to step away, and I knew she was right.

throw shot and discus, but we will keep it to ourselves how it went. Let's just say it was a big honor to us how interested they were in knowing what we do and how we train.

Later, the King of Sweden, Carl XVI Gustav, invited all Swedish Olympians to the castle for a celebration. It was a nice reunion of athletes that got to know each other at the Games because of the Covid restrictions. Everyone was called up on stage for recognition in front of the Royal Family, which was a huge honor.

It was a magic time, but exhausting on all of us, and as the 2022 season began, Daniel, Simon, and Fanny all struggled to find some rhythm.

Fanny threw 19.22m and got fourth at the Indoor Worlds, but it was her only competition over 19 meters indoors. The guys had a nice visit to Iceland for a discus competition in May hosted by my hometown of Selfoss, the Icelandic Federation, and my club, UMF Selfoss. Daniel threw 69.27m there and then 71.47m at Uppsala in June to take the world lead. But they could find no consistency, and at the same time Kristjan Čeh (now coached by Gerd) and Mykolas Alekna (the son of Gerd's former nemesis) both hit their stride.

And as my athletes struggled, so did I.

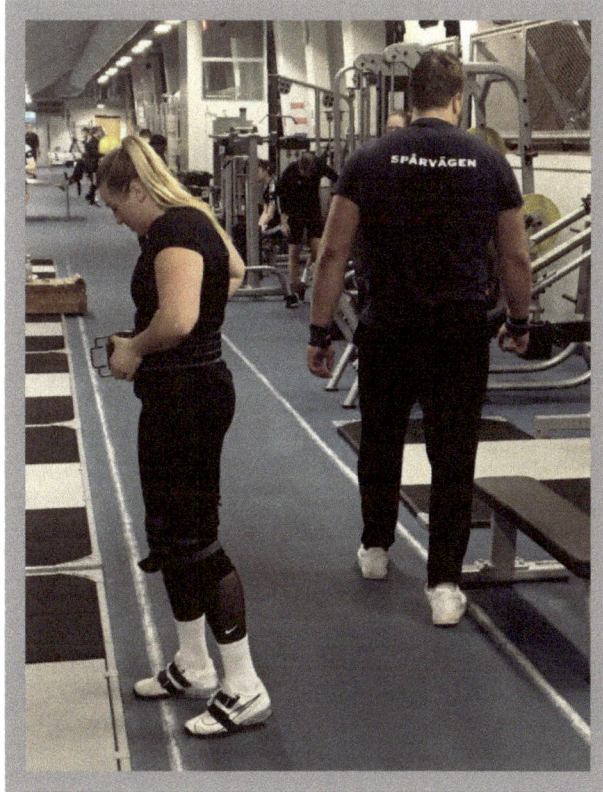

In the HPC in Växjö on a regular training day

My contract with the Swedish Olympic Committee called for me to consult with other coaches and to do lectures on coaching and training, and I began to feel the strain of combining those responsibilities with the full-time duties of a coach.

I had promised Anna that if I started to feel again like I did when I was hospitalized in 2016, I would make a change, and so after our training camp in Chula Vista in March, I dropped most of my consulting duties. The Swedish Olympic Committee was very supportive about this. My main job was to produce medals, and they did not want me distracted from that goal.

As the World Championships approached, I devoted all my energy to getting us ready, but life on the road was made even harder that summer when lots of people started traveling again after the Covid years. The situation at the airports in Europe became absolutely impossible, with lines of three or four hours any time you traveled. Several times during the early summer I had to get up at 3 a.m. only to arrive at the airport in Stockholm and see a line 200 meters long just to get into the terminal. Once, desperate to make my flight, I found a woman with three or four kids near the front of the line and pretended to be her husband. I started talking to her and playing with the kids and then I just stayed with them in line. She was probably thinking, "What in the hell is this man doing?" That's how crazy it was.

I felt drained as the time approached when we would travel to America for a pre-camp before the World Championships. The day before we were meant to leave, I was talking with Anna and with Henrik Gustafsson, the mental coach who works with my group, when Henrik asked me a strange question.

"Have you ever considered not going to the World Championships?"

"No," I replied. "I have not considered that."

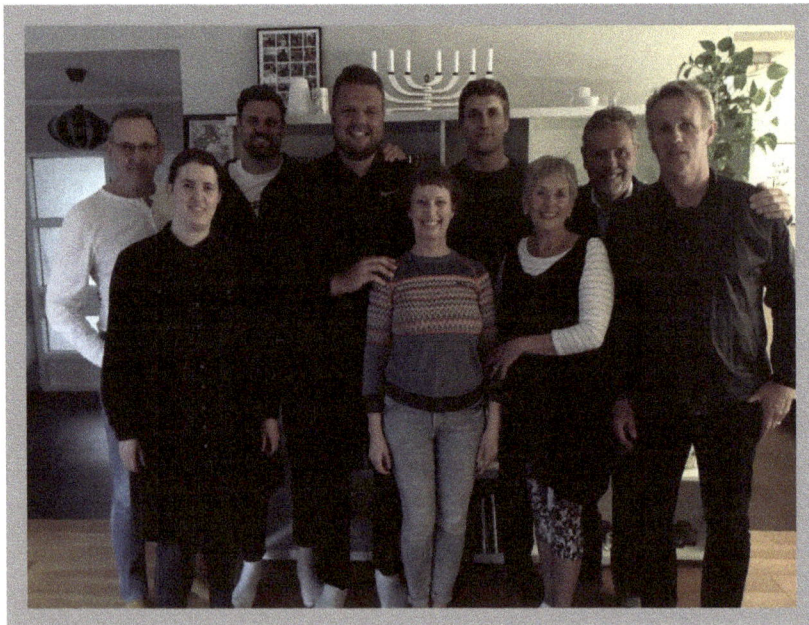

Icelandic Hospitality in Selfoss, Iceland. Left to right: Ólafur, husband of Aðalbjörg, my sister; Þóra, their daughter; Simon; Daniel; Aðalbjörg, my sister; Sven Martin; Hjördís, wife of my oldest brother Þorvaldur; Þorvaldur, and me.

"Well," he asked, "is it something you should consider?"

At any other time in my career, I would immediately have told Henrik, "No, stop bothering me with nonsense." But on this day, I sat in silence for thirty minutes while he and Anna waited for my answer.

My journey to that moment had begun many years ago in Selfoss. One day, as a young boy, I was delivering the evening newspaper after school, and I took a little break, sitting on my bicycle in the winter cold. I looked towards the mountain called Ingólfsfjall with its flat top and steep sides, rising up on the horizon a few kilometers away. Ingólfsfjall was named after Ingólfur Arnarson, the first Norse settler of Iceland, who came there in the year 874. His arrival is considered the birthday of our country. My friends and I would sometimes dress as American cowboys and ride our bikes to Ingólfsfjall to hide among the rocks and shoot at each other with toy pistols.

It was getting dark, and as I sat resting and breathing in the cold air, I could hear the Ölfusá river flowing through the town. It is a big river with a strong current, very beautiful and also very dangerous.

In those days, I knew the name of pretty much every family in Selfoss. Sitting on my bike, I could see the glow of lights through the windows of the houses, and I knew those families were going about their business, eating dinner or just relaxing after a day of work or school.

And at that moment I said to myself, "One day, every person in those houses is going to know me because of sports."

Fifty years later, sitting in the lobby of a hotel in Karlstad, Sweden, with Anna and Henrik, my vow had come true. I had competed in four Olympics and five World Championships as a discus thrower. During my career as a coach, my athletes had won many medals at international championships, including Olympic and World Championship golds for Gerd and Daniel.

That success made me famous in Iceland, just as I had dreamed. But there was a cost.

During all the years that Anna and I had been together, I was constantly on the road. Aside from 2020 when Covid made it hard to travel, I averaged 150 days away from home every year of my coaching career. That meant Anna, even when she was studying for her PhD and working herself, often had to manage raising our children without my help.

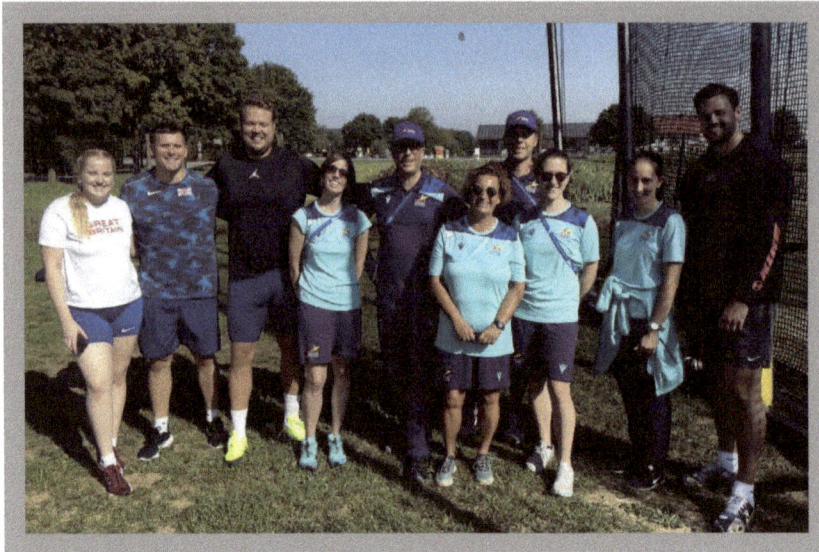

Making friends with volunteers at the EC in Munich

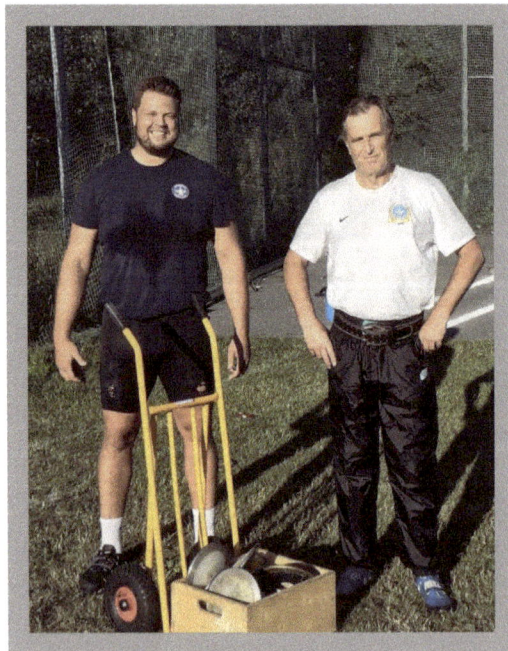

With Åke Ruus training at Sätra throwing field in Stockholm

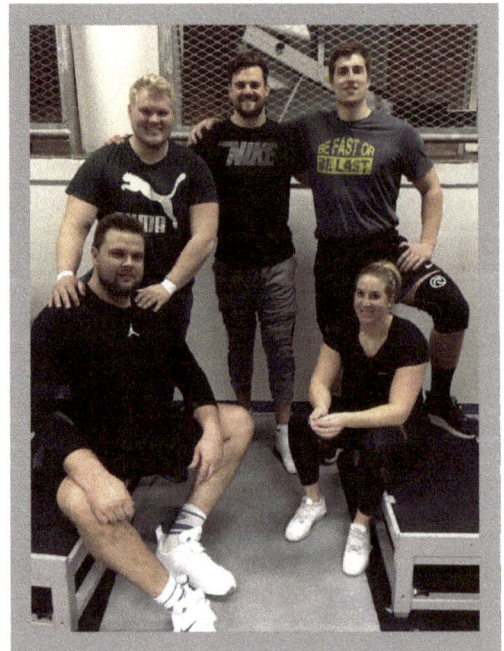

My Global Throwing group from 2020-2022

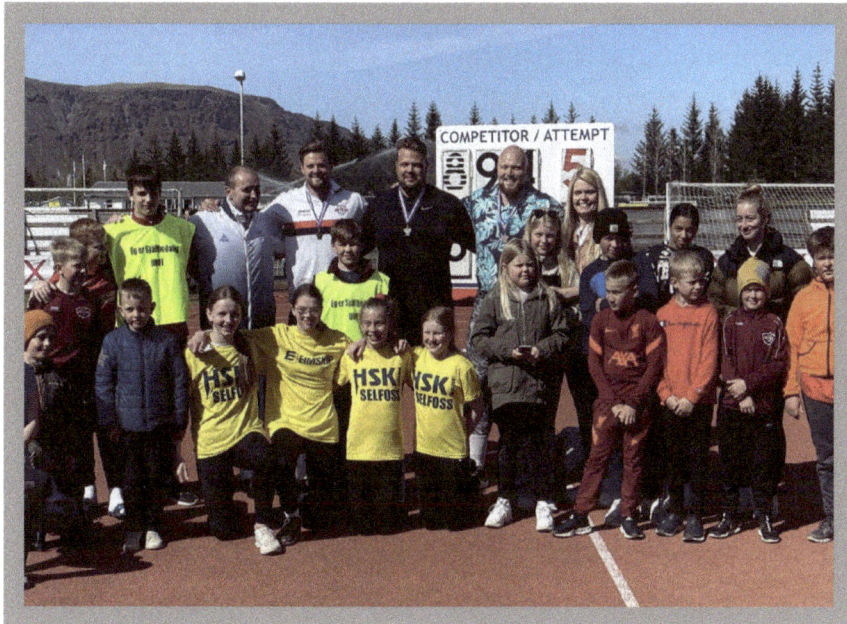

In Selfoss, Iceland with the Icelandic President Guðni Th. Jóhannesson along with Guðni Valur Guðnason the Icelandic discus thrower and Vala Flosadóttir, bronze medalist in women's pole vault at the Sydney OG in 2000.

And when I was not traveling, I was often so busy training my athletes that I would not arrive home until after Anna had put the children to bed. Then, when the pressure of getting the most out of Gerd or Daniel or Joachim Olsen would get to me, I'd wake up in the middle of the night to watch film and try to see if there was anything I was missing which might cost them their chance to win a medal.

In 2016, when I was hospitalized with panic attacks, a doctor asked me when was the last time I had a day off. I looked at my calendar and saw I had worked sixty-six days in a row. The panic attacks put an end to my streak, but as soon as I felt a little better, I went back to working the same kind of hours.

All that time, I knew I was risking my health, and even worse, I knew I was causing a lot of pain for Anna. But I was driven by the idea that if I was going to be a coach, I was going to do it the right way, and there could be no compromise.

Now the look on Anna's face as she waited for me to answer Henrik's question told me the time for compromise had come. I would stay home and not travel to the Worlds.

I did almost nothing for the next eighteen days, which was a PB for me. During the previous month when I'd felt exhausted, I'd had five incidents where I lost my temper—also a PB—but after a few days of rest I started to feel like myself again and to look forward to getting back to work when my group returned from the United States.

Anna and I had many serious talks during that break. We sometimes fought and sometimes cried, but when I asked her what was the highlight of our years together, she said this was it. This break, when we finally had time to sit and try to figure out what was best for the future.

I kept track of my athletes remotely while they were in America. It was disappointing that Daniel and Simon did not medal at the Worlds, but there were reasons for optimism. Daniel threw 70 meters in warmups and hit 69 meters in round three, which showed he was in great shape. But then, just like at the 2018 European Championships, his throw was ruled a foul after an official checked the video. Daniel could not overcome this bit of misfortune and ended up finishing fourth behind Kristjan Čeh, Mykolas Alekna, and his old nemesis Gudžius. Simon, as usual, was at his best on the big stage. He threw 68.11m in qualification–a season's best at the time–then 67.00m in the final, but it was not enough to get a medal. He ended up fifth. Kristjan broke the World Championships record with a throw of 71.13m, which made me very proud of Gerd.

Marcus finished tenth in Eugene, and Fanny eleventh, so we took no medals there, and none later that summer at the European Championships either, when Simon finished fourth and Daniel fifth, Marcus ninth and Fanny fourth.

For the 2022 season, my group had four fourth-place finishes, two fifth-place finishes, one ninth, one tenth, and one eleventh-place finish at international championships. Compared to what we achieved in 2021—Olympic gold and silver, European Indoor silver—you could say that we had a terrible year. But I do not look at it that way.

As I said, a professional thrower cannot make excuses for a poor performance. It is their job to compete well, regardless of the conditions. Bad weather. Bad officials. A stadium full of noisy people where you cannot hear yourself think. A stadium full of no people where you can hear someone sneeze one hundred meters away. None of that matters.

But after a competition, it is the coach's job to evaluate the performance realistically. All of us would like for our athletes to win the gold medal every time, but you will not last long in this business if you are ready to jump from a bridge when they finish second or fourth or thirteenth. Instead, a coach must always look for the positive. Were Marcus and

Mac Wilkins
on Daniel's future

66 I believe that Daniel can still throw a PB. Certainly, things are different for his body now than five years ago, but everyone's career has its own timetable, and Daniel is strong and still has the best technique among the big guys, so I don't think he's missed his window of opportunity.

The world record is not out of the question but having that as a goal in the discus is too heavy of a burden for even the best throwers to take on. So much of it comes down to having the right wind conditions. Jürgen Schult had a monster wind when he set the record in 1986, and I don't see Daniel going around chasing big winds.

In 2022, two big waves named Čeh and Alekna came crashing down on the beach, and maybe in the end they will make a high-water mark higher than Daniel, which will be a mental challenge for him but also give him all the more reason to focus on what he is doing. He will have to deal with their results and not let it be a drag on him.

With Vésteinn retiring, Daniel will have to look at his situation now and find a perspective to move forward, and I think he will. 99

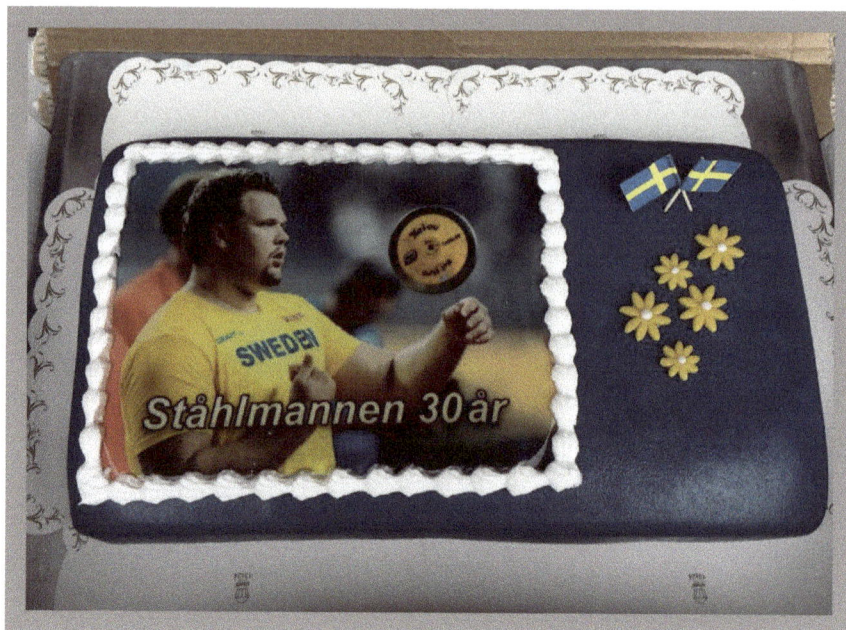

Daniel turned 30 on the 27th of August at the meet in Helsingborg and was rewarded by a friend Thomas Lindell with this cake.

Fanny capable of finishing higher than tenth and eleventh at the World Championships? Certainly. But for both, it was their best finish ever at a Worlds. Was Simon happy with fourth place in Eugene after winning the silver medal at the Olympics? No, but the 68.11m he threw in qualification was his best distance ever in a major championship. Was it disappointing for Daniel to finish the 2022 season with no medals? Yes, but he is healthy and strong and still young enough to contend in 2023 and 2024.

Consider the career of Gerd Kanter. After the 2008 Olympic Games, he did not take another gold medal. In 2009, he had a huge disappointment at the World Championships where he was expected to win but ended up finishing third. Should he have retired and gone to live in a cave after that? He probably considered it for a couple of days. But it was my job to remind him that the sun would come up tomorrow and there were many discus throwers in the world—including those who finished fourth and fifth in Berlin—who would have been delighted to trade places with him.

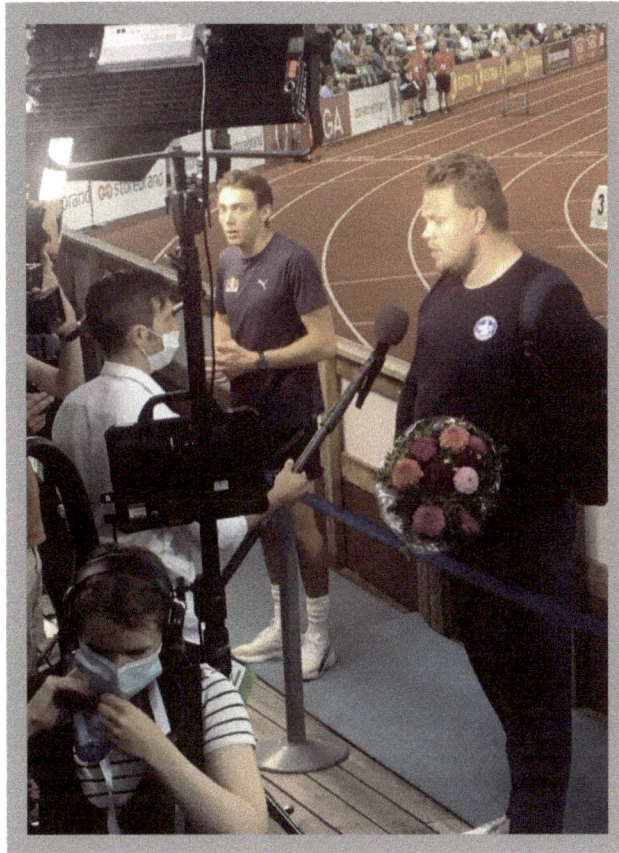

Two Swedish Olympic Champions

Instead of throwing himself into the Spree River, Gerd went back to work and over the rest of his career took two more World Championships medals, three more European Championships medals, and an Olympic bronze in 2012 when, after struggling the entire year, he produced a season's best 68.03m in the final. None of this would have happened if he did not learn to take something positive from a disappointing result.

And staying positive was not as hard as you might think for my group after the 2022 season. After all, Marcus made the finals at the European and World Championships, which was a big breakthrough for him. Fanny hit a PB and national record of 19.42m in August. Simon broke 70 meters for the first time in his career when he threw 70.42m to win the Swedish Championships. And Daniel produced the world-leading throw (71.47m) for the seventh year in a row.

Also, even though Daniel turned thirty last summer, Joe Kovacs showed old guys can still get it done when he hit a PB of 23.23m at the Diamond League final at the age of 33.

So, when the 2022 season ended, I was optimistic about our prospects moving forward.

Then, on October 6th, I received an opportunity from the Icelandic Sports and Olympic Association. They proposed a five-year contract for the position of Head of Elite Sports in Iceland with a mission to build a strong developmental system for school kids all the way up to the elite level.

If I accepted the position, it would be the final phase of my career. Anna and I would move to Iceland for the duration of the contract, then we would retire to our country house in Sweden.

It would get me off the road, but it would mean giving up active coaching. I would have to say goodbye to my group.

Anna and I considered the offer for three months then finally decided to take it. She was very happy, and so was I, though it was not easy telling my athletes. To their credit, they were extremely understanding and supportive, even though parting ways after we'd been through so much together was tough.

But once I got through those conversations and helped get them set up with new situations and new coaches, I felt a huge relief. Soon, I began to feel that Vésteinn Hafsteinsson the person—not just the coach—was back. I had missed him!

It was very emotional for Daniel and me when I told him of my decision. As you now know, we had been through a lot together. As our meeting ended, he said to me, "Well, this must be your dream come true!"

And he was right. The little kid from Selfoss had grown up to be a success on the international stage. Now, it was time to go home.

Looking back, I hope that my throwers, Daniel and Gerd and all the others, somehow made a small difference in the world.

I know this might seem silly. In a time when there is war and many people do not have enough to eat, what does it matter who wins a medal at the Olympic Games?

Kajsa Bergqvist
on Daniel's impact on Swedish Athletics

"Daniel and I come from almost the same place in the northern suburbs of Stockholm. To see him develop from being a big, strong, puppy with all this power and ability to become the great person and sportsman that he is today has been a fantastic journey.

With his talent and personality, he became a star and made discus into Sweden's national sport. I was working as a television commentator when Daniel started to get big, and I knew that because of him all the Swedish people would be watching the discus, so I always had to be prepared. Before each broadcast, I googled every result and statistic about how many throwers had been over 70 meters the most times in a season or who had the best all-time top ten average. I felt like I was becoming a professor of the discus!

And Swedish throwing is booming now. It has become our best discipline. When I was an athlete, jumps was where we had the most success. There was me and Stefan Holm, and Christian Olsson and Carolina Klüft. We were a proud jumping nation, but it feels like throwing has taken over that position. We have three women shot putters who might make the final in the 2023 World Championships, and we have some excellent young discus girls coming up.

This is because a whole group of young boys and girls was inspired by Daniel and Simon and Fanny. Young people looked at how those three succeeded and said to themselves, "If I train like them and take the sport seriously like them, I could be a champion someday, too."

"I think he can throw very far again. After the Olympic Games, he got a little bit mentally tired because his focus had been on Tokyo and the Olympics for so many years, so I think he had trouble feeling the same energy in 2022. When I saw him on the television, I could see he has not the same focus as earlier. It is much easier to perform if you love to be there and feel the energy. If you don't feel that, it is not so easy.

And this was a normal human reaction. After so many hard years of work, you need a break to find new goals and new energy.

But Daniel loves to be a discus thrower, and I think now that he is in a new environment with a new coach he can find the energy, and if he does, he can throw as far as he wants to."

I will answer with a story. After Gerd won gold in 2008, there was a huge celebration in Tallinn. The streets were packed with people. After the ceremonies ended, we were walking through the crowd when a young man stopped and asked me to step aside with him. He took me to meet two old ladies in babushkas who had come to the celebration. They were poor and had clearly suffered through the difficult years of the Second World War and the Soviet occupation of their country. The young man introduced us, and each of the ladies handed me a single red rose. It was their way of thanking me for coaching Gerd. His achievement filled them with pride and happiness and allowed them, at least for a little while, to forget how hard life could be.

Raul often talked about the power of sports to unite people and bring them joy, and at that moment, I knew he was right.

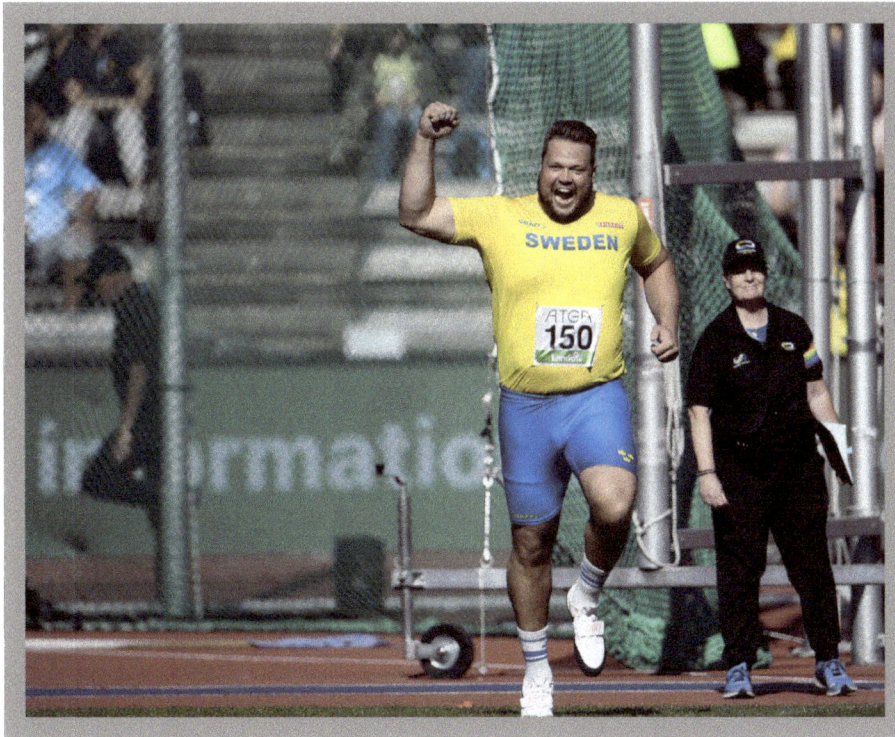

Daniel on one of his famous runs

It was similar in Sweden when Daniel and Simon won their medals at the Olympics. After the dark days of the pandemic, people had a reason to laugh.

I believe that Daniel, Simon, Fanny and Marcus will bring people more joy as they continue their careers with new coaches. As for me, I will do my best to help my home country produce its own sports heroes.

Maybe somewhere in Iceland right now there is a kid with smooth moves playing hockey or basketball or high jumping or throwing the discus who just needs the right coach to tap them on the shoulder and say, "I think you could be good at this. Let's take the journey together."

And maybe, in a few years, I'll stand and watch as we have a celebration in Reykjavík and a coach receives his own red rose. That day, my heart will be full.

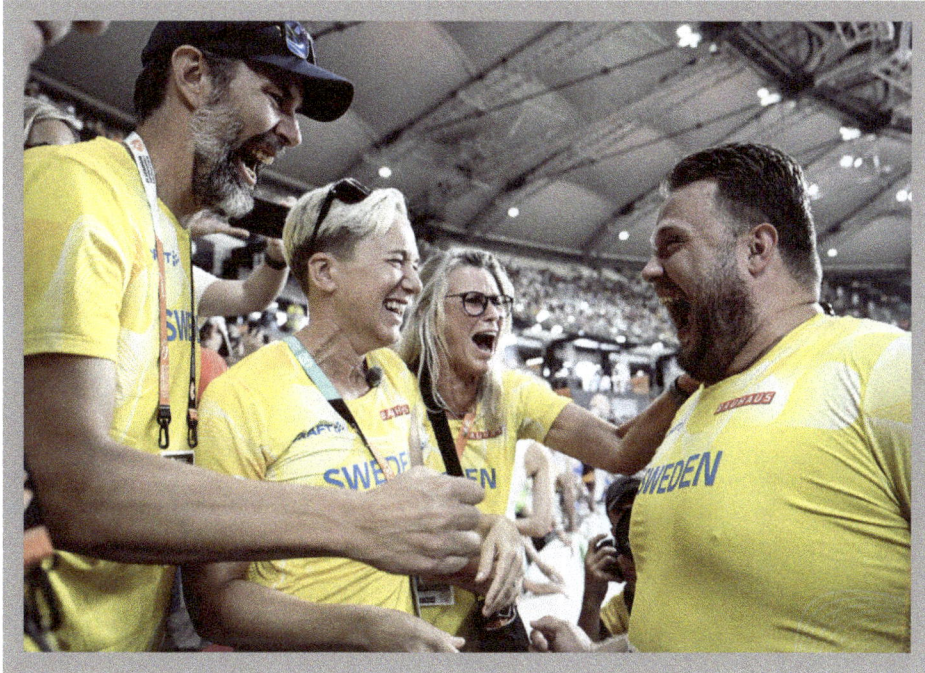

Staffan Jönsson, Team Sweden head coach Kajsa Bergqvist, Team Sweden coordinator Petra Ericson, and Daniel after his stunning triumph in Budapest.

Epilogue

Putting a book into its final shape is not a simple matter, but as this past summer wore on, we got closer and closer to having a finished product. The words were written, and all that remained was to secure the rights to all the photos we wished to use and to have the words and pictures laid out in a pleasing format.

Then Daniel made the greatest throw in World Championships history.

Before I stepped away from coaching last March, I tried to help my athletes find the best possible situation going forward. With my help and with the support of the Norwegian Federation, Marcus was able to join a group coached by my old friend Paolo Dal Soglio, who has had great success with the shot putters Zane Weir and Leonardo Fabbri. Simon wished to move back to his hometown of Sixarby, which would put him close to the training facilities of the Upsala IF Athletics Club, managed by Henrik Wennberg. I've known Henrik for a long time. He competed in two European Championships and one World Championships as a shot putter, and also threw the discus 62.56m, and I was happy when he agreed to coach Simon.

Fanny and Daniel ended up moving to Malmö to train with Staffan Jönsson, the 2005 Swedish champion in the discus. Staffan has had a career in banking while at the same time coaching the shot putter Wictor Petersson, who was World U20 silver medalist in 2016 and four-time Swedish champion. I did my best to mentor him over the years, and he and Wictor were often together with my group at different training camps, so Fanny and Daniel already knew Staffan and liked him. One day in January of 2023, they called and asked him to be their coach, and after he got over his surprise, he said yes.

Staffan has picked my brains more than any young coach over the years, so he already knew everything about how my planning and periodization worked. After he agreed to take on Fanny and Daniel, I sent him my training plans from last year and this year and gave him advice about what I felt they needed to focus on physically, mentally, and technically.

At the same time, I wanted Staffan to put his stamp on their training, and he did this in a very smart way. He did not change much, but put little things of himself in there.

I told Staffan that at thirty years old, Daniel was not going to get faster and would not be able to change his technique too much. The main thing he needed to do was to feel good and have fun throwing the discus again.

In 2022, our final season together, Daniel had a hard time when Kristjan Čeh knocked him off the top of the ladder. It started right away when Daniel threw 65.97m at the Diamond League meeting in Birmingham and Kristjan threw 71.27m. Kristjan also beat him at the Diamond League meetings in Rabat, Rome, and Stockholm, then took over the World title in Eugene with a Championships record throw of 71.13m.

Daniel beat Kristjan in Turku, and ended the season having the world-leading throw for the seventh time in a row, but I could tell something was bothering him all summer. When the season ended, he finally admitted to me that he hated being stepped over by Kristjan and also by Mykolas Alekna, who got second at Worlds and was European champion.

When I sat down with Staffan last spring, I told him I think we have a golden chance with Daniel in 2023. I believed that Daniel was over being upset about Kristjan, and if he was, he could go into the season letting Kristjan feel all the pressure and just have fun.

And that is exactly what happened. Daniel was happy living in Malmö, and Staffan did a great job keeping him feeling fresh with his training. Also, Staffan speaks with

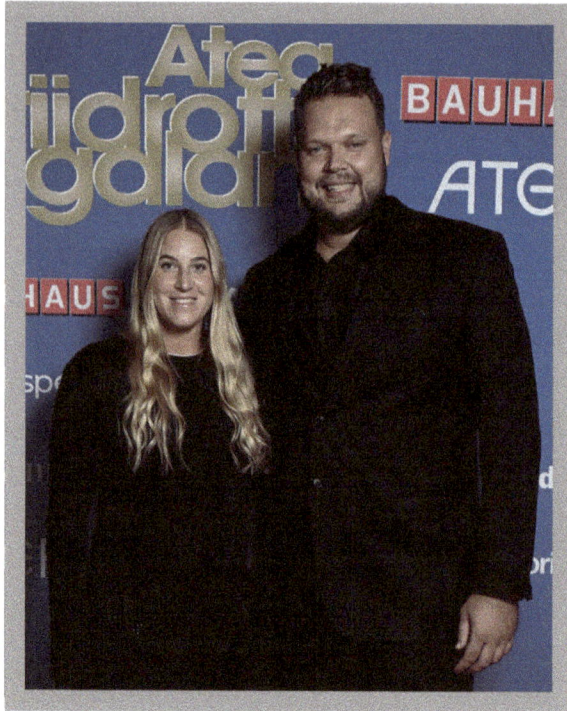

Fanny and Daniel at Friidrottsgalan 2023, the annual
awards ceremony for Swedish Athletics.

the accent of the southern Swedish people, which Daniel gets a big kick out of, so every
time Staffan opened his mouth it made Daniel happy.

It seemed right away that Daniel was feeling better this year when he threw 69.21m
in May at the Diamond League meeting in Rabat. Kristjan still beat him, but the 69.21m
was farther than Daniel threw at any Diamond League meeting during 2022.

Then Daniel went 70.38m to beat Kristjan in Turku, Finland. At their next meeting—
the Heino Lipp Memorial in Estonia—Kristjan won with a throw of 71.86m to Daniel's
71.45m, the longest second-place throw in history.

It was great to see Daniel throwing far and competing well against Kristjan, but it
was important for him to also do this outside of his comfort zone of Sweden and Finland.
He finally did in July when he defeated Kristjan at both the Gyulai István Memorial
in Hungary and the Diamond League meeting in London with throws of 68.98m
and 67.03m.

Going into the World Championships, I still considered Kristjan the favorite with Daniel likely to take the silver medal.

It was a good sign when Daniel had the best throw in qualification in Budapest, but then he did not look comfortable on his first three throws in the final. His second attempt of 66.58m was enough to keep him in the top eight, but Kristjan was still way ahead at 69.27m.

Then, in round four, Daniel threw 69.37m to take the lead.

That put a lot of pressure on Kristjan, and he showed the heart of a champion by hitting 70.02m on his final attempt to put himself back in the lead. But at major championships, they revise the order before the sixth round so the one leading the competition gets the final say. Because Daniel had been in first place after five rounds, he would now have a chance to answer Kristjan.

Daniel's 69.37m was already farther than he had ever thrown in a Worlds or Olympics, and he told me later he felt no weight on his shoulders when he walked into the ring. He was just going to step in and go for it.

He threw 71.46m, a new World Championships record, and under the circumstances—having to beat 70.02m on his final attempt—I would say the greatest clutch throw in discus history.

Looking ahead, I believe Daniel has a good chance to take a medal at the 2024 Olympics, and who knows after that? If he and Staffan are smart about his training like they were in 2023, there is no reason he cannot be competitive for a few years more.

I was incredibly proud of Daniel's performance in Budapest. As you know from reading this book, it was never easy for Daniel to be in the spotlight, and for him to respond at the biggest moment on the biggest stage was amazing. Even better, Daniel seems to be extremely happy being together with Fanny in Malmö. I know he will be a great husband someday, and probably the best father on Earth, and that is more important than all the medals he has ever won.

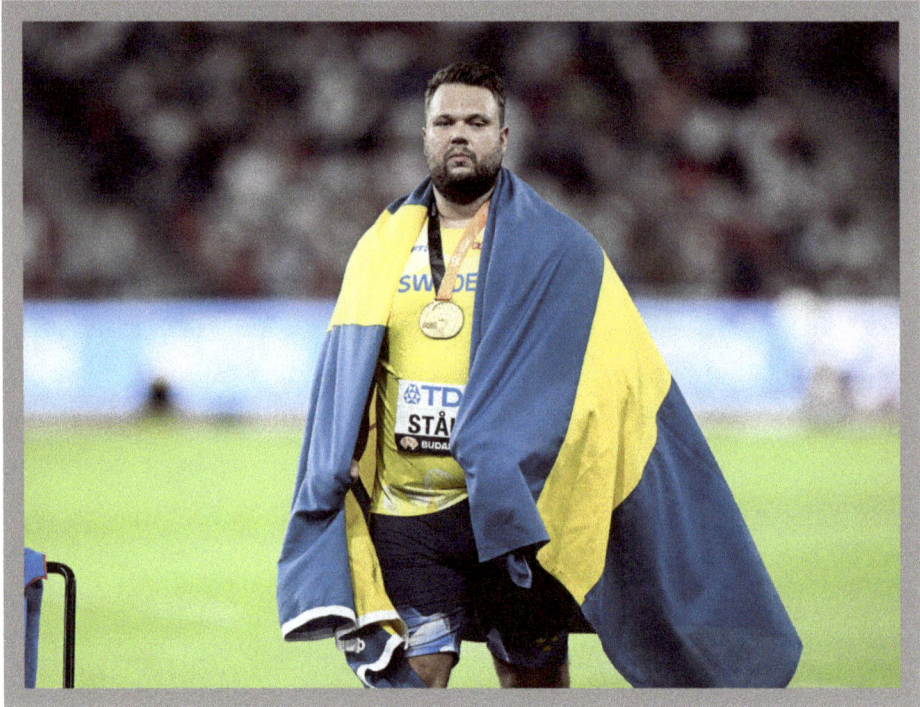

Daniel took his second World Championships gold in Budapest with the greatest clutch throw in discus history.

ABOUT THE AUTHORS

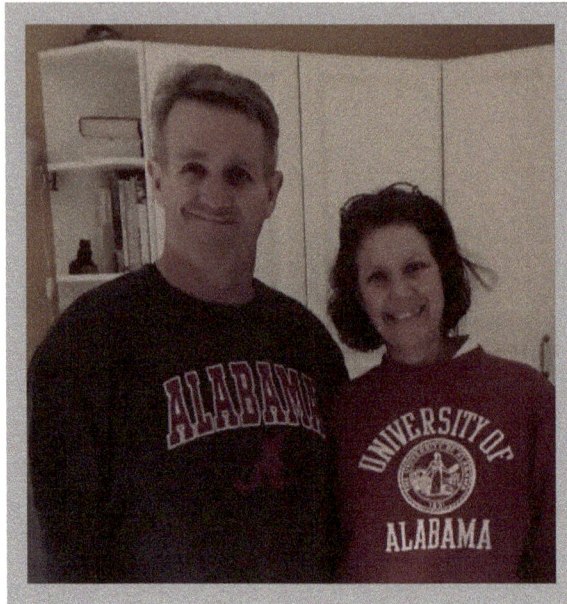

Roll Tide Roll

Vésteinn Hafsteinsson is one of the most successful throwing coaches in history. A proud son of Selfoss, Iceland, Vésteinn competed in four Olympic Games and five World Championships as a discus thrower. After transitioning to coaching in the mid 1990's, he worked with 56 athletes from 10 different countries, most prominently Joachim Olsen of Denmark (2004 Olympic shot put silver), Gerd Kanter of Estonia (2007 World and 2008 Olympic discus gold), and Fanny Roos (2021 European Indoor shot put silver, 2023 bronze), Simon Pettersson (2021 Olympic discus silver), and Daniel Ståhl (2019 World and 2021 Olympic discus gold) of Sweden. In total, Vésteinn's athletes earned 20 medals at major international championships. He and his wife, Anna, have raised three children—Örn, Olga and Albert—and plan to spend the next five years in Iceland where Vésteinn will serve as Head of Elite Sports.

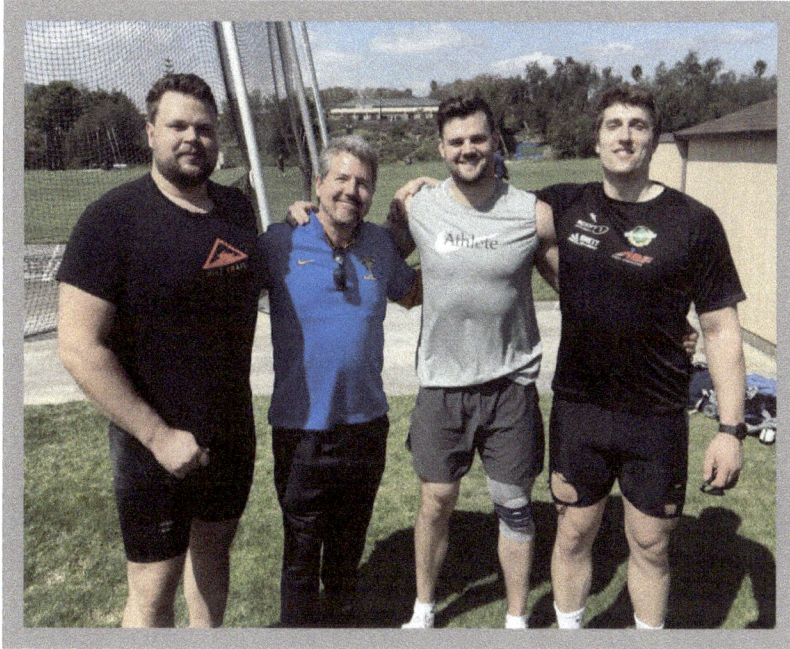

Dan McQuaid with the guys in Chula Vista in the spring of 2022

Dan McQuaid is a high school throwing coach and retired English teacher who lives with his immensely patient wife in the Chicago suburb of Naperville, Illinois. He has two grown stepsons and a nine-year-old grandson who regularly destroys him in driveway basketball. Dan is proud that his daughter, KC, has embarked on her own career as a teacher, coach, and writer, though why she chose distance running after having been raised among large people with chalky hands remains a mystery. Dan and Roger Einbecker, who also contributed to this book, manage the Mcthrows.com website, through which they produce articles and webinars about the sport of throwing.

APPENDIX

*The information contained in this table came from
the Swedish T&F Performance data base
(https://www.friidrottsstatistik.se/atswe.php?Sex=1&ID=112326)
and the World Athletics data base
(https://worldathletics.org/athletes/sweden/daniel-stahl-14375325).*

Statistics courtesy of Priit Tänava

Table 1

Detailed Comparison of Daniel Stahl's Performances in 2017 vs 2016									
2016						Series average	First 3 attempt avg	Last 3 attempt avg	
Average Distance	62.10	63.78	62.30	62.00	64.14	63.55	62.98	62.73	63.23
Good Attempt	65%	57%	43%	50%	31%	81%	55%	55%	54%
Over 63m	13%	22%	9%	13%	19%	44%	20%	14%	25%

2017						Series average	First 3 attempt avg	Last 3 attempt avg	
Average Distance	63.69	65.17	66.06	64.27	64.65	65.08	64.82	64.97	64.67
Good Attempt	65%	75%	58%	58%	67%	72%	66%	66%	66%
Over 63m	25%	60%	47%	37%	33%	44%	41%	44%	38%

	Round in Which Best Throw Occurs					
	Rnd 1	Rnd 2	Rnd 3	Rnd 4	Rnd 5	Rnd 6
2016	17%	17%	17%	0%	13%	35%
2017	5%	30%	10%	10%	20%	25%

Table 2

Dist	PL	Meet	Location	Date	Series					
					Rnd 1	Rnd 2	Rnd 3	Rnd 4	Rnd 5	Rnd 6

DANIEL STÅHL'S 2011 ANNUAL COMPETITIVE PERFORMANCES

Dist	PL	Meet	Location	Date	Rnd 1	Rnd 2	Rnd 3	Rnd 4	Rnd 5	Rnd 6
2011 Season (1.75 kg)										
56.84 i	1		Växjö	13.3.11						
57.68	1		Sätra/K	7.5.11						
60.85	1		Bålsta	14.5.11						
53.69	10	Werfertage U20	Halle, GER	21.5.11						
NMQ	-	European Junior Champs	Tallinn, EST	23.7.11						
55.60	5	Swedish Championships	Gävle/R	13.8.11						
58.64	1	Swedish Junior Champs	Velinge	27.8.11						
57.66	1	Nordic Junior Champs	Copenhagen, DEN	4.9.11						
55.25	1		Huddinge/J	18.9.11						
53.00Q	4		Helsingborg	24.9.11						
57.70	1		Helsingborg	24.9.11						

Table 3

| Dist | PL | Meet | Location | Date | Series | | | | | |
					Rnd 1	Rnd 2	Rnd 3	Rnd 4	Rnd 5	Rnd 6
DANIEL STÅHL'S 2012 ANNUAL COMPETITIVE PERFORMANCES										
55.75i	1		Växjö	10.3.12						
57.45	3	European Cup Winter Throw	Bar, MNE	17.3.12	53.45	X	54.30	57.22	X	57.45
56.20	27	Triton Invitational	La Jolla, CA	26.4.12						
54.36	10	Triton Invitational	La Jolla, CA	28.4.12						
55.13	10	Chula Vista OTC Pre-Oly	Chula Vista, CA	3.5.12						
55.65	6	Oxy Invite	Eagle Rock, CA	5.5.12						
54.09	6	Hallesche Werfertage U23	Halle, GER	20.5.12						
54.00	3		Nyköping	26.5.12						
52.76	7	BIGBANK Kuldliiga	Tartu, EST	29.5.12						
58.67	2		Tallinn, EST	3.6.12						
57.83	1	Helsingborg Throws Meet U23	Helsingborg	9.6.12						
57.93	1	Helsingborg Throws Meet U23	Helsingborg	10.6.12						
58.41	1	Bottnaryd Throwing Meet	Bottnaryd	16.6.12						
57.88	1	Helsingborg Throws Meet U23	Helsingborg	17.6.12						
57.14	1	Uppsala Uppsalaspelen	Uppsala	30.6.12						
56.82	11	BIGBANK Kuldliiga	Viljandi, EST	3.7.12						
57.32	10	Sollentuna GP	Sollentuna	5.7.12						
57.77	1		Sätra/K	12.7.12						
56.15	1		Sätra/K	15.7.12						
61.42	2	Nordic-Baltic U23 Champs	Jessheim, NOR	22.7.12						
59.98	1	Västeras Gurkspelen	Västerås/Ap	4.8.12						
56.23	3		Stockholm/S	7.8.12						
62.16	2	Swedish Championships	Stockholm/S	25.8.12	61.11	X	62.16	61.38	X	61.03
59.29	3	Göteborg SWE-FIN Match	Gothenburg/U	2.9.12	58.86	59.29	X	55.24	X	55.22
59.70	6	IAAF World Challenge	Zagreb, CRO	4.9.12						
60.25	8	Kose ERGO World Games	Kose, EST	13.9.12	56.02	60.25	X	X	57.14	58.05
58.65	1		Sätra/K	16.9.12						

Table 4

Dist	PL	Meet	Location	Date	Series					
					Rnd 1	Rnd 2	Rnd 3	Rnd 4	Rnd 5	Rnd 6
56.86 i	3	Cougar Invitational	Provo, UT	10.1.13						
56.67	7	European Cup Winter Throw	Castellón, ESP	16.3.13	X	X	X	56.67	55.62	X
53.53	5	Soka Peace Invitational	Aliso Viejo, CA	20.4.13						
54.66	15	Triton Invitational	La Jolla, CA	25.4.13						
56.11	11	Triton Invitational	La Jolla, CA	27.4.13						
54.91	2	Hulst Pinkster Atletiekgala	Hulst, NED	20.5.13						
60.74	2	Tartu Gustav Sule Memorial	Tartu, EST	28.5.13	54.66	59.04	X	X	56.03	60.74
54.36	9	Bislett Games DL	Oslo, Norway	13.6.13	54.36	X	X			
57.77	2	Göteborg Kvilles Vårtävling	Gothenburg/S	14.6.13						
58.61	6	Sollentuna Folksam GP	Sollentuna	27.6.13	58.61	X	X	55.36	54.96	X
56.39	4	Bottnaryd Throwing Meet	Bottnaryd	29.6.13						
58.19	2		Växjö/A	2.7.13						
59.83	4	Helsingborg Öresundsspelen	Helsingborg	7.7.13						
57.44Q	7	European U23 Championships	Tampere, FIN	11.7.13	56.96	57.44	56.10			
61.29	4	European U23 Championships	Tampere, FIN	13.7.13	X	59.51	58.93	X	61.29	58.85
59.59	8	Luzern Spitzen Leichtathletik	Lucerne, SUI	17.7.13	57.95	59.59	X	X	X	X
57.44	2	Hässleholm HAIS-spelen	Hässleholm	28.7.13						
59.50	1	Göteborg Night of Athletics	Gothenburg	31.7.13						
58.74	1	Mölndal Folksam Challenge	Mölndal	3.8.13						
59.30	1	Swedish U23 Championships	Västerås	11.8.13						
60.47	1	Umea Folksam Challenge	Umeå	18.8.13						
NM	-	DN Gala DL	Stockholm/S	22.8.13	X	X	X			
59.07	2	Swedish Championships	Borås	31.8.13	58.88	58.21	59.07	X	X	X
58.30	3	Finnkampen	Stockholm/S	7.9.13	58.30	57.65	X	X	56.52	X
58.46	1		Sätra/K	22.9.13						

DANIEL STÅHL'S 2013 ANNUAL COMPETITIVE PERFORMANCES

Table 5

DANIEL STÅHL'S 2014 ANNUAL COMPETITIVE PERFORMANCES

Dist	PL	Meet	Location	Date	Series					
					Rnd 1	Rnd 2	Rnd 3	Rnd 4	Rnd 5	Rnd 6
60.09i	1	v3Nat	Tampere, FIN	8.2.14	57.62	58.48	57.65	60.09	X	54.77
57.70	2	European Cup Winter Throw	Leiria, POR	15.3.14	X	56.40	57.70	56.66	X	57.61
58.49 i	3		Växjö/Tue	22.3.14						
64.30	3	Chula Vista HP/OTC Series	Chula Vista, CA	24.4.14	X	64.30	61.66	58.98	58.00	62.10
63.09	3	Triton Invitational	La Jolla, CA	26.4.14	63.09	54.91	57.50	55.53	X	X
66.89	1	Steve Scott Invitational	Irvine, CA	3.5.14	63.48	66.89	X	X	59.54	61.00
60.68	1	København	Copenhagen, DEN	10.5.14	X	60.68	X	55.13	X	54.96
59.34	2	Werfertage	Halle, GER	18.5.14	57.13	X	59.25	X	X	59.34
62.60	1	Lokeren Grote Prijs	Lokeren, BEL	24.5.14	55.53	60.78	X	62.60	60.62	55.62
62.05	8	Golden Gala DL	Rome, Italy	5.6.14	57.29	62.05	58.64	60.18	60.73	X
62.62	3	Iberoamericano de Atletismo	Huelva, ESP	12.6.14	61.77	X	60.98	62.11	62.62	60.12
57.24	11	European Team Champs	Braunschweig, GER	22.6.14	X	57.24	57.12			
60.28	4	Sollentuna Folksam GP	Sollentuna	26.6.14	59.07	60.28	X	58.44	59.84	X
63.02	1	Bottnaryd Throwing Meet	Bottnaryd	28.6.14	X	X	60.73	59.63	63.02	58.69
63.54	1	Göteborg	Gothenburg/SK	30.6.14	60.30	60.50	X	X	62.31	
64.60	5	Lausanne Athletissima DL	Lausanne, SUI	3.7.14	60.66	63.55	60.73	X	64.60	60.62
60.60	1	Swedish Club Championships	Borås	5.7.14	X	58.35	X	60.60		
61.60	7	Monaco Herculis	Monaco, MON	18.7.14	61.60	61.42	X	X	X	61.37
63.61	1	Nordic-Baltic U23 Champs	Copenhagen, DEN	27.7.14	X	62.03	59.64	60.25	63.61	X
63.69	1	Swedish Championships	Umeå	2.8.14	61.64	X	57.06	X	63.69	X
59.01Q	24	European Championships	Zurich, SUI	12.8.14	X	56.51	59.01			
60.96	7	Birmingham GP DL	Birmingham, GBR	24.8.14	59.56	X	X	X	X	60.96
61.77	1	Finnkampen	Helsinki, FIN	30.8.14	X	60.36	61.77	58.63	60.26	59.16
57.80	1	Castorama	Växjö/A	2.9.14						

Table 6

Dist	PL	Meet	Location	Date	Rnd 1	Rnd 2	Rnd 3	Rnd 4	Rnd 5	Rnd 6
					Series					
60.37	1	Folksam GP	Uppsala	7.6.15	X	X	X	X	55.96	60.37
61.23	2	Tartu Gustav Sule Memorial	Tartu, EST	9.6.15	X	61.23	X	X	X	X
60.55	2	European Athletics Festival	Bydgoszcz, POL	14.6.15	60.55	59.64	X	X	X	X
NM	-	European Team Champs	Cheboksary, RUS	21.6.15	X	X	X			
62.93	1	Sollentuna Folksam GP	Sollentuna	25.6.15	X	60.16	X	X	X	62.93
62.85	2	Bottnaryd Throwing Meet	Bottnaryd	27.6.15	X	59.57	X	62.85	X	X
57.87	4		Helsingborg	28.6.15						
63.38	1	Swedish Club Championships	Sundsvall	1.7.15	59.26	61.04	63.38	57.10	58.00	62.18
60.26	2		Madrid, ESP	11.7.15	X	58.42	58.90	X	60.26	59.56
60.77	7	Luzern Spitzen Leichtathletik	Lucerne, SUI	14.7.15	60.07	X	X	60.77	59.50	59.87
62.76	2	Valter Kalami Memorial	Viljandi, EST	19.7.15	60.56	58.58	X	62.76	61.83	X
63.03	5	Bauhaus DL	Stockholm/S	30.7.15	61.25	X	X	X	60.75	63.03
58.94	4		Helsingborg	3.8.15	58.59	58.94	55.97	56.45	X	58.15
60.20	3	Swedish Championships	Söderhamn	8.8.15	59.39	X	60.20	X	X	X
63.20	1		Gothenburg/SK	10.8.15	X	X	60.19	X	X	63.20
60.48	2	Göteborg Folksam GP	Gothenburg/S	14.8.15	56.45	58.03	56.83	60.39	58.25	58.68
61.12	1	Umea Folksam Challenge	Umeå	16.8.15	58.58	X	X	59.91	61.12	X
62.66Q	9	IAAF World Championships	Beijing, CHN	27.8.15	62.66	61.22	62.06			
64.73	5	IAAF World Championships	Beijing, CHN	29.8.15	61.74	60.42	64.42	64.73	X	X
59.05	2	Göteborg Folksam GP	Gothenburg/S	5.9.15	59.05	X	X	X	X	X
NM	-	ISTAF	Berlin, GER	6.9.15	X	X	X			
62.21	1	Finnkampen	Stockholm/S	12.9.15	61.86	59.34	X	X	61.64	62.21

DANIEL STÅHL'S 2015 ANNUAL COMPETITIVE PERFORMANCES

Table 7

Dist	PL	Meet	Location	Date	Series					
					Rnd 1	Rnd 2	Rnd 3	Rnd 4	Rnd 5	Rnd 6
61.09i	1	BothniaG	Mustasaari, FIN	6.2.16	60.32	61.09	59.59	59.93	X	57.12
56.84 i	7	ISTAF	Berlin, GER	13.2.16	X	X	X	X	X	56.84
66.74	1	Spring Fling	Salinas, CA	17.4.16						
66.42	2	Triton Invitational	La Jolla, CA	23.4.16	64.93	66.42	X	X	X	65.20
64.72	1	Steve Scott Invitational	Irvine, CA	30.4.16	X	63.21	X	63.52	64.72	X
64.06	4	IAAF Diamond League	Doha, Qatar	6.5.16	X	64.06	X			
61.09	3	Mohammed VI d'Athletisme	Rabat, MAR	22.5.16	61.09	X	X			
63.25	4	Golden Gala DL	Rome, Italy	2.6.16	62.11	63.25	60.46			
61.93	7	Birmingham GP DL	Birmingham, GBR	5.6.16	60.80	X	61.93			
63.68	1	Tartu Gustav Sule Memorial	Tartu, EST	13.6.16	X	62.24	X	X	63.05	63.68
63.47	1	Bauhaus-Galan	Stockholm/S	16.6.16	X	X	X	59.05	63.47	X
62.86	3	Umea Folksam Challenge	Umeå	21.6.16	62.61	X	X	X	X	62.86
63.42	1	Sollentuna Folksam GP	Sollentuna	28.6.16	63.42	X	59.12	X	X	X
65.78Q	2	European Championships	Amsterdam, NED	7.7.16	X	X	65.78			
64.77	5	European Championships	Amsterdam, NED	9.7.16	62.17	64.04	X	X	62.53	64.77
62.87	2	Monaco Herculis	Monaco, MON	15.7.16	61.96	62.20	X	X	X	62.87
66.92	2	Gyulai István Memorial	Székesfehérvár, HUN	18.7.16	63.13	66.28	65.27	X	66.92	66.34
64.24	1	Karlstad Folksam GP	Karlstad	27.7.16	61.09	X	X	61.59	X	64.24
62.26Q	14	Olympic Games	Rio de Janeiro	12.8.16	60.78	X	62.26			
64.76	1	Helsingborg Folksam GP	Helsingborg	21.8.16	59.84	62.64	62.59	60.32	X	64.76
68.72	1	Swedish Championships	Sollentuna	28.8.16	X	65.09	X	63.83	X	68.72
65.46	1	Finnkampen	Tampere, FIN	3.9.16	65.46	64.15	60.19	65.00	X	64.74
65.78	1	Van Damme Memorial	Brussels, BEL	9.9.16	X	64.53	65.78	62.73	X	64.01
61.80	1		Sätra/K	14.9.16	61.80	X	X			

The table title is: **DANIEL STÅHL'S 2016 ANNUAL COMPETITIVE PERFORMANCES**

Table 8

Dist	PL	Meet	Location	Date	Series					
					Rnd 1	Rnd 2	Rnd 3	Rnd 4	Rnd 5	Rnd 6
66.90i	1	Nordenkampen	Tampere, FIN	11.2.17	X	X	X	57.89	66.90	X
61.51	4	European Throwing Cup	Las Palmas, ESP	11.3.17	X	X	X	61.51	X	X
68.36	1	Hartnell Spring Fling	Salinas, CA	21.4.17	X	68.36	X	67.02	X	66.33
68.11	1	Hartnell Spring Fling	Salinas, CA	22.4.17	62.29	59.69	67.11	X	67.44	68.11
63.87	1	Steve Scott Invitational	Irvine, CA	29.4.17	62.49	63.87	61.00	63.48	61.89	60.08
64.14	3	IAAF Diamond League	Shanghai, CHN	13.5.17	61.03	63.87	64.14	X	63.76	60.48
68.07	1	Werfertage	Halle, GER	20.5.17	64.57	X	X	65.30	68.07	66.94
64.44	3	FBK Games	Hengelo, NED	11.6.17	X	63.74	X	64.44	X	63.58
68.06	1	Bislett Games	Oslo, Norway	15.6.17	62.60	64.95	67.36	65.36	62.58	68.06
68.13	2	Bauhaus-Galan	Stockholm/S	18.6.17	66.25	67.34	66.88	X	66.95	68.13
66.41	1	European Team Champs	Vaasa, FIN	25.6.17	X	66.41	X	65.63		
71.29	1	Sollentuna Folksam GP	Sollentuna	29.6.17	68.88	X	71.29	X	X	62.83
67.59	1	Swedish Team Champs	Borås	7.7.17						
66.73	1	Müller Anniversary Games	London, GB	9.7.17	65.63	63.59	66.23	X	65.19	66.73
65.64 i	1		Växjö/Tue	20.7.17	62.53	X	65.36	X	65.64	64.42
67.26	1	Karlstad Folksam GP	Karlstad	25.7.17	64.11	66.07	65.47	65.35	58.64	67.26
67.64Q	1	IAAF World Championships	London, GB	4.8.17	61.83	67.64				
69.19	2	IAAF World Championships	London, GB	5.8.17	X	69.19	66.58	68.57	X	63.06
67.80	1	Swedish Championships	Helsingborg	25.8.17	58.33	66.99	65.23	X	67.80	X
64.18	7	Van Damme Memorial	Brussels, BEL	1.9.17	X	64.18	X	X	60.96	X
67.37	1	Finnkampen	Stockholm/S	3.9.17	67.37	61.68	X	62.44	X	X
62.26	1	Castorama	Karlstad/M	9.9.17						

Table 9

Dist	PL	Meet	Location	Date	Series					
					Rnd 1	Rnd 2	Rnd 3	Rnd 4	Rnd 5	Rnd 6

DANIEL STÅHL'S 2018 ANNUAL COMPETITIVE PERFORMANCES

Dist	PL	Meet	Location	Date	Rnd 1	Rnd 2	Rnd 3	Rnd 4	Rnd 5	Rnd 6
66.81	1	European Throwing Cup	Leiria, POR	10.3.18	66.81	64.96	X	X	60.63	X
68.03	2	Chula Vista Throws	Chula Vista, CA	12.4.18	64.43	64.24	X	59.62	68.03	X
64.98	4	Triton Invitational	La Jolla, CA	14.4.18	62.69	64.06	64.98	X	62.44	64.94
64.35	3	Long Beach Invitational	Long Beach, CA	21.4.18	63.60	61.68	63.15	X	X	64.35
63.16	2	Steve Scott Invitational	Irvine, CA	28.4.18	X	X	63.16	X	62.56	X
66.65	2	Werfertage	Halle, GER	26.5.18	X	X	63.01	X	62.49	66.65
64.84	4	Golden Gala	Rome, Italy	31.5.18	62.31	64.56	64.51	63.80	64.10	64.84
67.04	3	Bislett Games	Oslo, Norway	7.6.18	X	66.55	X	X	60.30	67.04
66.16	6	Bauhaus-Galan	Stockholm/S	10.6.18	66.16	64.46	X	X	X	X
67.39	1	Bottnaryd Throwing Meet	Bottnaryd	16.6.18	66.62	X	67.39	X	65.73	65.11
66.17	1	Sollentuna Folksam GP	Sollentuna	28.6.18	66.17	X	65.20	65.23	64.11	63.85
60.46	12	Meeting de Paris	Paris, FRA	30.6.18	X	60.46	X			
64.46	4	Gyulai István Memorial	Székesfehérvár, HUN	2.7.18	64.46	63.89	X	63.96	X	60.87
68.12	1	Team Championship	Helsingborg	6.7.18	65.26	66.74	68.12	X	65.68	64.12
69.11	1	Karlstad Folksam GP	Karlstad	25.7.18	X	X	66.31	69.11	X	X
67.07Q	1	European Championships	Berlin, GER	7.8.18	67.07					
68.23	2	European Championships	Berlin, GER	8.8.18	X	X	64.20	68.23	X	X
NM	-	Göteborg Folksam GP	Gothenburg/S	18.8.18	X	X	X	X	X	X
69.72	1	Swedish Championships	Eskilstuna	26.8.18	64.91	X	67.48	65.88	69.72	X
66.74	3	Van Damme Memorial	Brussels, BEL	31.8.18	65.59	64.63	X	65.86	66.74	63.35
68.00	1	Finnkampen	Tampere, FIN	1.9.18	68.00	62.70	X	65.92	65.86	X
64.84	5	IAAF Continental Cup	Ostrava, CZE	8.9.18	64.84	X	X			
64.91	1		Tallinn, EST	13.9.18	X	64.91	63.14	64.84		
66.00	3		Sätra/K	17.9.18	64.16	X	66.00	65.38		

Table 10

DANIEL STÅHL'S 2019 ANNUAL COMPETITIVE PERFORMANCES

Dist	PL	Meet	Location	Date	Rnd 1	Rnd 2	Rnd 3	Rnd 4	Rnd 5	Rnd 6
					Series					
70.56	1	IAAF Diamond League	Doha, Qatar	3.5.19	69.63	70.49	70.56	69.54	69.50	70.32
69.57	1	Bauhaus-Galan	Stockholm/S	30.5.19	X	69.57	X	69.33	X	X
NM	-	Paavo Nurmi Games	Turku, FIN	11.6.19	X	X	X			
69.94	2	Mohammed VI	Rabat, MAR	16.6.19	X	67.84	X	69.94	X	X
69.12	1	Sollentuna Folksam GP	Sollentuna	18.6.19	68.52	X	69.12	X	X	X
69.89	1	Team Championship	Helsingborg	26.6.19	68.59	66.63	69.89	X	X	X
71.86	1	Bottnarydskastet	Bottnaryd	29.6.19	68.76	68.83	69.71	X	71.86	X
68.93	1	Karlstad GP	Karlstad	3.7.19	67.22	X	68.88	67.28	68.93	67.92
68.77	1	Gyulai István Memorial	Székesfehérvár, HUN	9.7.19	X	67.61	66.40	68.77	X	68.51
70.89	1	Varberg GP	Varberg	15.7.19	67.99	68.79	70.78	70.36	70.89	70.37
68.56	1	Müller Anniv Games	London, GB	21.7.19	62.77	66.61	68.56	X	X	65.71
61.38	3	Team EC Super L	Bydgoszcz, POL	11.8.19	X	61.38	X	X		
69.42	1	Finnkampen	Stockholm/S	25.8.19	69.42	69.39	X	X	X	X
69.23	1	Swedish Championships	Karlstad	31.8.19	69.08	69.23	67.67	X	66.49	X
68.68	1	Van Damme Memorial	Brussels, BEL	6.9.19	68.68	67.66	68.32	64.73	67.49	67.36
67.88Q	1	IAAF World Champs	Doha, Qatar	28.9.19	X	67.88				
67.59	1	IAAF World Champs	Doha, Qatar	30.9.19	66.59	67.18	67.59	65.83	X	67.05

Table 11

					Series					
DANIEL STÅHL'S 2020 ANNUAL COMPETITIVE PERFORMANCES										
Dist	**PL**	**Meet**	**Location**	**Date**	**Rnd 1**	**Rnd 2**	**Rnd 3**	**Rnd 4**	**Rnd 5**	**Rnd 6**
65.92	1	Impossible Games	Oslo, Norway	11.6.20	X	X	64.92	X	65.92	X
NM	-	Kringelkastet	Södertälje	14.6.20	X	X	X	X	X	X
70.25	1	Victor Svanesohn Mem	Helsingborg	21.6.20	66.35	65.25	70.25	68.34	68.41	63.62
64.92	1	Bottnarydskastet	Bottnaryd	27.6.20	64.92	62.65	63.86	64.05	X	63.18
66.55	1	Västerortsmästerskapen	Hässelby	4.7.20	X	66.45	66.55	66.42	X	X
68.10	1	Karlstad GP	Karlstad	8.7.20	68.10	63.50	65.95	66.07	X	64.45
68.72	1	Kasttävling	Växjö/A	12.7.20	67.56	X	64.81	64.74	68.72	66.38
68.48	1	Kuortane Games	Kuortane, FIN	1.8.20	X	65.91	67.51	68.48	X	66.70
68.10	1	Team Championship	Gothenburg/S	6.8.20	X	X	68.07	X	X	68.10
71.37	1	Sollentuna Folksam GP	Sollentuna	10.8.20	68.38	X	71.37	X	X	X
69.23	1	Paavo Nurmi Games	Turku, FIN	11.8.20	X	X	69.23	X	X	X
68.74	1	Swedish Championships	Uppsala	15.8.20	65.26	X	X	X	68.74	X
67.31	1	Gyulai István Memorial	Székesfehérvár, HUN	19.8.20	66.52	65.17	X	67.31	66.67	X
69.17	1	Bauhaus-Galan	Stockholm/S	23.8.20	X	69.17	67.36	67.44	X	68.57
69.20	1	Finnkampen	Tampere, FIN	5.9.20	66.95	X	69.20	X	69.01	65.94
67.28	1	Skolimowska Memorial	Chorzów, POL	6.9.20	66.54	X	67.01	X	66.55	67.28
66.42	1	Golden Spike	Ostrava, CZE	8.9.20	63.90	66.01	66.42	X	X	66.00
65.89	2	ISTAF	Berlin, GER	13.9.20	X	65.89	X	X	65.88	X
68.87	1	Hanžeković Memorial	Zagreb, CRO	15.9.20	66.97	68.87	67.55	68.87	67.16	X
68.54	1	Castorama	Hässelby	17.9.20	68.30	68.54	67.03	X		

Table 12

Dist	PL	Meet	Location	Date	Series					
					Rnd 1	**Rnd 2**	**Rnd 3**	**Rnd 4**	**Rnd 5**	**Rnd 6**
NMi	-	Diskustävling	Växjö	7.3.21	X	X	X	X	X	X
69.71	1	Victor Svanesohn Mem	Helsingborg	22.5.21	69.71	X	X	67.94	69.04	X
69.11	2	Kasttävling	Växjö/A	29.5.21	X	X	X	X	69.11	X
66.81	1	Göteborg Friidrott GP	Gothenburg/S	2.6.21	X	66.81	X	X	X	X
68.11	1	Paavo Nurmi Games	Turku, FIN	7.6.21	66.26	X	65.86	68.11	66.93	X
68.03	1	Sollentuna GP	Sollentuna	13.6.21	65.95	67.25	66.52	68.03	X	X
67.64	1	Karlstad GP	Karlstad	22.6.21	67.22	65.18	67.64	X	66.48	X
70.55	1	Kuortane Games	Kuortane, FIN	26.6.21	63.61	X	69.99	70.21	X	70.55
68.65	1	Team Championship	Halmstad	29.6.21	67.78	X	67.48	68.65	68.13	68.51
68.65	1	Bislett Games	Oslo, Norway	1.7.21	67.26	65.52	66.95	67.17	68.65	65.72
68.64	1	Bauhaus-Galan	Stockholm/S	4.7.21	67.33	X	X	68.64	X	68.23
67.71	1	Gyulai István Memorial	Székesfehérvár, HUN	6.7.21	65.20	65.45	67.71	X	X	65.44
71.40	1	Bottnarydskastet	Bottnaryd	10.7.21	70.27	71.40	X	64.67	X	X
66.12Q	1	XXXII Olympics Games	Tokyo, JPN	30.7.21	66.12					
68.90	1	XXXII Olympics Games	Tokyo, JPN	31.7.21	63.72	68.90	65.16	66.10	67.03	64.58
67.04	1	Swedish Championships	Borås	28.8.21	64.53	66.79	67.04	66.09	X	63.80
69.31	1	Van Damme Memorial	Brussels, BEL	1.9.21	69.31	X	X	X	68.59	67.01
69.09	1	Finnkampen	Stockholm/S	5.9.21	64.08	69.09	X	65.95	68.98	66.83
66.49	1	Diamond League Final	Zurich, SUI	9.9.21	66.49	X	X	X	65.64	X
67.79	1	Hanžeković Memorial	Zagreb, CRO	14.9.21	67.79	64.12	X	X	X	66.29
68.02	1	Tjalves diskustävling	Norrköping	17.9.21	63.02	X	X	68.02	X	64.27

Table title: DANIEL STÅHL'S 2021 ANNUAL COMPETITIVE PERFORMANCES

Table 13

Dist	PL	Meet	Location	Date	Series					
					Rnd 1	Rnd 2	Rnd 3	Rnd 4	Rnd 5	Rnd 6
67.62	1i	Diskustävling	Växjö	25.02.22	66.85	x	67.62	x	x	x
65.95	2	EP-w (21)	Leiria	12.03.22	61.90	x	65.95	x	64.12	x
69.11	1	CVEATC Discus Inv	Chula Vista, CA	07.04.22	67.45	66.67	66.80	69.11	x	x
68.44	1	Triton Inv	La Jolla, CA	09.04.22	66.17	67.01	x	x	x	68.44
67.65	1	MSR (62)	Walnut, CA	16.04.22	65.72	66.30	67.65	x	65.92	66.96
65.97	3	British GP/DL	Birmingham	21.05.22	65.86	65.97	x	x	65.52	x
69.27	1	Selfoss Classic	Selfoss	28.05.22	x	65.81	66.62	67.01	69.27	64.65
67.16	2	Mohammed VI/DL	ar-Rabāṭ	05.06.22	64.35	67.16	66.94	66.26	66.58	62.53
65.87	3	Golden Gala (42)/DL	Roma	09.06.22	65.68	63.85	65.87	x	x	x
68.97	1	Sollentuna / Folksam GP	Sollentuna	12.06.22	66.00	67.40	64.42	65.29	67.50	68.97
70.62	1	PNG (60)	Turku	14.06.22	70.62	x	x	67.75	64.55	x
66.26	1	Motonet GP	Kuortane	18.06.22	x	66.26	x	65.43	64.29	x
71.47	1	Club Ch	Uppsala	21.06.22	67.05	x	71.47	69.51	x	68.15
69.22	1	Bottnarydskastet	Bottnaryd	25.06.22	x	67.33	x	65.75	x	69.22
67.57	3	Bauhaus (56)/DL	Stockholm	30.06.22	x	63.90	x	65.03	67.57	66.16
66.75	1	Karlstad / Folksam GP	Karlstad	03.07.22	66.75	x	x	65.29	x	x
65.95Q	7	WCh (18) - Q (66.00)	Eugene, OR	17.07.22	x	65.95	x			
67.10	4	WCh (18)	Eugene, OR	19.07.22	66.59	65.99	x	65.39	67.10	66.86
70.29	2	NC (127) (SWE Ch)	Norrköping	06.08.22	68.67	68.37	68.97	66.54	70.29	69.07
67.01	3	Gyulai (12)	Székesfehérvár	08.08.22	66.55	66.74	66.84	67.01	x	66.32
66.39Q	3	ECh (25) - Q (66.00)	München	17.08.22	66.39	-	-			
66.39	5	ECh (25)	München	19.08.22	66.39	65.80	64.76	63.42	65.94	66.00
67.72	1	Victor Svanesohn Memorial	Helsingborg	27.08.22	64.87	66.16	x	x	x	67.72
65.34	1	FIN v SWE	Helsinki	03.09.22	64.90	64.94	65.34	x	x	x
65.16	5	Weltklasse/DL	Zürich	08.09.22	62.88	x	x	x	65.16	61.47
64.93	5	Hanžeković (72)	Zagreb	11.09.22	x	64.93	x	x	x	x

Table 14

Dist	PL	Meet	Location	Date	Series					
					Rnd 1	Rnd 2	Rnd 3	Rnd 4	Rnd 5	Rnd 6
67.14	2	Diamond/DL	Doha	05.05.23	64.31	x	67.14	64.32	63.97	65.85
69.01	1	Tjalves Diskusgala	Norrköping	18.05.23	68.62	x	67.52	69.01	x	x
69.21	2	MohammedVI/DL	ar-Rabāṭ	28.05.23	64.77	64.89	67.53	69.21	x	68.2
70.93	1	Sollentuna / Folksam GP	Sollentuna	11.06.23	68.24	67.09	x	68.16	70.93	x
70.38	1	PNG (61)	Turku	13.06.23	64.21	x	65.43	67.6	70.38	69.63
71.45	2	Heino Lipp (15)	Jõhvi	16.06.23	66.28	x	x	67.2	x	71.45
67.25	1	ETC	Chorzów	24.06.23	67.25	x	x	x	x	x
67.57	2	Bauhaus (57)/DL	Stockholm	02.07.23	x	67.57	x	x	x	x
70.25	1	Karlstad / Folksam GP	Karlstad	05.07.23	67.36	66.88	70.25	x	x	x
69.8	1	LAG-SM	Sollentuna	08.07.23	64.17	x	69.8	x	66.87	x
68.98	1	Gyulai (13)	Székesfehérvár	18.07.23	66.3	68.98	x	x	x	x
67.03	1	DL/London Athletics Meet	London	23.07.23	x	64.89	x	67.03	x	x
64.67Q	1	NC (128) (SWE Ch) - Q	Söderhamn	28.07.23	64.67	-	-			
67.61	1	NC (128) (SWE Ch)	Söderhamn	29.07.23	67.61	67.1	x	x	66.84	x
67.3	1	Folksam GP	Malmö	05.08.23	67.3	x	x	65.89	x	66.13
65.22	1	Victor Svanesohn Memorial	Helsingborg	07.08.23	x	x	x	65.22	x	x
66.25Q	1	WCh (19) - Q (66.50)	Budapest	19.08.23	64.58	66.25	64.99			
71.46	1	WCh (19)	Budapest	21.08.23	63.01	66.58	x	69.37	67.56	71.46
66.89	2	Tallinn 2023	Tallinn	31.08.23	63.05	64.5	66.89	65.46	64.24	65.27
66.44	1	SWE v FIN	Stockholm	02.09.23	x	x	65.35	x	66.44	66.4
67.24	1	Galà dei Castelli	Bellinzona	04.09.23	63.97	67.24	63.02	62.72	62.17	x
67.36	3	Prefontaine/DL	Eugene, OR	17.09.23	64.59	67.13	67.36	x	x	65.62

The table title spans: **DANIEL STÅHL'S 2023 ANNUAL COMPETITIVE PERFORMANCES**

Table 15

				Rnd 1	Rnd 2	Rnd 3	Rnd 4	Rnd 5	Rnd 6	

Daniel Ståhl All Time Performances as of 31.10.2023										
#	Mark	Date	Competition	Rnd 1	Rnd 2	Rnd 3	Rnd 4	Rnd 5	Rnd 6	series avg
1	71.86	6/29/19	Bottnarydskastet, Bottnaryd, Bottnaryd	68.76	68.83	69.71	x	71.86	x	69.790
2	71.47	6/21/22	Club Ch, Uppsala	67.05	x	71.47	69.51	x	68.15	69.045
3	71.46	8/21/23	WCh (19), Budapest	63.01	66.58	x	69.37	67.56	71.46	67.596
4	71.45	6/16/23	Heino Lipp (15), Jõhvi	66.28	x	x	67.2	x	71.45	68.310
5	71.40	7/10/21	Bottnarydskastet, Bottnaryd	70.27	71.40	x	64.67	x	x	68.780
6	71.37	8/10/20	Sollentuna / Folksam GP, Sollentuna	68.38	x	71.37	x	x	x	69.875
7	71.29	6/29/17	Sollentuna / Folksam GP, Sollentuna	68.88	x	71.29	x	x	62.83	67.667
8	70.93	6/11/23	Sollentuna / Folksam GP, Sollentuna	68.24	67.09	x	68.16	70.93	x	68.605
9	70.89	7/15/19	Varberg / Folksam GP, Varberg	67.99	68.79	70.78	70.36	70.89	70.37	69.863
10	70.62	6/14/22	PNG (60), Turku	70.62	x	x	67.75	64.55	x	67.640
11	70.56	5/3/19	Diamond/DL, Doha	69.63	70.49	70.56	69.54	69.50	70.32	70.007
12	70.55	6/26/21	Motonet GP, Kuortane	63.61	x	69.99	70.21	x	70.55	68.590
13	70.38	6/13/23	PNG (61), Turku	64.21	x	65.43	67.6	70.38	69.63	67.450
14	70.29	8/6/22	NC (127) (SWE Ch), Norrköping	68.67	68.37	68.97	66.54	70.29	69.07	68.652
15	70.25	6/21/20	Helsingborg	66.35	65.25	70.25	68.34	68.41	63.62	67.037
16	70.25	7/5/23	Karlstad / Folksam GP, Karlstad	67.36	66.88	70.25	x	x	x	68.163
17	69.94	6/16/19	Mohammed VI/DL, ar-Rabāṭ	x	67.84	x	69.94	x	x	68.890
18	69.89	6/26/19	Club Ch, Helsingborg	68.59	66.63	69.89	x	x	x	68.370
19	69.80	7/8/23	LAG-SM, Sollentuna	64.17	x	69.8	x	66.87	x	66.947
20	69.72	8/26/18	NC (123) (SWE Ch), Eskilstuna	64.91	x	67.48	65.88	69.72	x	66.998
21	69.71	5/22/21	Victor Svanesohn, Helsingborg	69.71	x	x	67.94	69.04	x	68.897
22	69.57	5/30/19	Bauhaus (53)/DL, Stockholm	x	69.57	x	69.33	x	x	69.450
23	69.42	8/25/19	SWE v FIN, Stockholm	69.42	69.39	x	x	x	x	69.405
24	69.31	9/1/21	VD (45)/DL, Bruxelles	69.31	x	x	x	68.59	67.01	68.303
25	69.27	5/28/22	Selfoss Classic, Selfoss	x	65.81	66.62	67.01	69.27	64.65	66.672
26	69.23	8/31/19	NC (124), Karlstad	69.08	69.23	67.67	x	66.49	x	68.118
27	69.23	8/11/20	PNG (58), Turku	x	x	69.23	x	x	x	69.230
28	69.22	6/25/22	Bottnarydskastet, Bottnaryd	x	67.33	x	65.75	x	69.22	67.433
29	69.21	5/29/23	MohammedVI/DL, ar-Rabāṭ	64.77	64.89	67.53	69.21	x	68.2	66.920
30	69.20	9/5/20	FIN v SWE, Tampere	66.95	x	69.20	x	69.01	65.94	67.775
31	69.19	8/5/17	WCh (16), London	x	69.19	66.58	68.57	x	63.06	66.850
32	69.17	8/23/20	Bauhaus (54)/DL, Stockholm	x	69.17	67.36	67.44	x	68.57	68.135
33	69.12	6/18/19	Sollentuna / Folksam GP, Sollentuna	68.52	x	69.12	x	x	x	68.820
34	69.11	7/25/18	Karlstad / Folksam GP, Karlstad	x	x	66.31	69.11	x	x	67.710
35	69.11	5/29/21	Kasttävling, Växjö	x	x	x	x	69.11	x	69.110
36	69.11	4/7/22	CVEATC Discus Inv, Chula Vista, CA	67.45	66.67	66.80	69.11	x	x	67.508
37	69.09	9/5/21	SWE v FIN, Stockholm	64.08	69.09	x	65.95	68.98	66.83	66.986
38	69.01	5/18/23	Tjalves Diskusgala, Norrköping	68.62	x	67.52	69.01	x	x	68.383
39	68.98	7/18/23	Gyulai (13), Székesfehérvár	66.3	68.98	x	x	x	x	67.640
40	68.97	6/12/22	Sollentuna / Folksam GP, Sollentuna	66.00	67.40	64.42	65.29	67.50	68.97	66.597
41	68.93	7/3/19	Karlstad / Folksam GP, Karlstad	67.22	x	68.88	67.28	68.93	67.92	68.046
42	68.90	7/31/21	Oly Games, Tōkyō	63.72	68.90	65.16	66.10	67.03	64.58	65.915
43	68.87	9/15/20	Hanžeković (70), Zagreb	66.97	68.87	67.55	66.41	67.16	x	67.392
44	68.77	7/9/19	Gyulai (9), Székesfehérvár	x	67.61	66.40	68.77	x	68.51	67.823
45	68.74	8/15/20	NC (125) (SWE Ch), Uppsala	65.26	x	x	x	68.74	x	67.000
46	68.72	8/28/16	NC (121) (SWE Ch), Sollentuna	x	65.09	x	63.83	x	68.72	65.880
47	68.72	7/12/20	Växjö	67.56	x	64.81	64.74	68.72	66.38	66.442

Table 15 (continued from previous page)

#	Mark	Date	Competition	Rnd 1	Rnd 2	Rnd 3	Rnd 4	Rnd 5	Rnd 6	series avg
			Daniel Ståhl All Time Performances as of 31.10.2023							
48	68.68	9/6/19	VD (43)/DL, Bruxelles	68.68	67.66	68.32	64.73	67.49	67.36	67.373
49	68.65	6/29/21	Laxaspelen, Halmstad	67.78	x	67.48	68.65	68.13	68.51	68.110
50	68.65	7/1/21	Bislett/DL, Oslo	67.26	65.52	66.95	67.17	68.65	65.72	66.878
51	68.64	7/4/21	Bauhaus (55)/DL, Stockholm	67.33	x	x	68.64	x	68.23	68.067
52	68.56	7/21/19	Anniversary Games/DL, London	62.77	66.61	68.56	x	x	65.71	65.913
53	68.54	9/17/20	Castorama, Hässelby	68.30	68.54	67.03	x			67.957
54	68.48	8/1/20	Motonet GP, Kuortane	x	65.91	67.51	68.48	x	66.70	67.150
55	68.44	4/9/22	Triton Inv, La Jolla, CA	66.17	67.01	x	x	x	68.44	67.207
56	68.36	4/21/17	Spring Fling Elite, Salinas, CA	x	68.36	x	67.02	x	66.33	67.237
57	68.23	8/8/18	ECh (24), Berlin	x	x	64.20	68.23	x	x	66.215
58	68.13	6/18/17	Bauhaus (51)/DL, Stockholm	66.25	67.34	66.88	x	66.95	68.13	67.110
59	68.12	7/6/18	Interclubs Final, Helsingborg	65.26	66.74	68.12	x	65.68	64.12	65.984
60	68.11	4/22/17	Spring Fling Open, Salinas, CA	62.29	59.69	67.11	x	67.44	68.11	64.928
61	68.11	6/7/21	PNG (59), Turku	66.26	x	65.86	68.11	66.93	x	66.790
62	68.10	7/8/20	Karlstad / Folksam GP, Karlstad	68.10	63.50	65.95	66.07	x	64.45	65.614
63	68.10	8/6/20	Club Ch, Göteborg	x	x	68.07	x	x	68.10	68.085
64	68.07	5/20/17	Werfertage (43), Halle (Saale)	64.57	x	x	65.30	68.07	66.94	66.220
65	68.06	6/15/17	Bislett/DL, Oslo	62.60	64.95	67.36	65.36	62.58	68.06	65.152
66	68.03	4/12/18	CV Throws - Elite, Chula Vista, CA	64.43	64.24	x	59.62	68.03	x	64.080
67	68.03	6/13/21	Sollentuna / Folksam GP, Sollentuna	65.95	67.25	66.52	68.03	x	x	66.938
68	68.02	9/17/21	Norrköping	63.02	x	x	68.02	x	64.27	65.103
69	68.00	9/1/18	FIN v SWE, Tampere	68.00	62.70	x	65.92	65.86	x	65.620
70	67.88	9/28/19	WCh (17) - Q (65.50), Doha	x	67.88	-				67.880
71	67.80	8/25/17	NC (122) (SWE Ch), Helsingborg	58.33	66.99	65.23	x	67.80	x	64.588
72	67.79	9/14/21	Hanžeković (71), Zagreb	67.79	64.12	x	x	x	66.29	66.067
73	67.72	8/27/22	Victor Svanesohn, Helsingborg	64.87	66.16	x	x	x	67.72	66.250
74	67.71	7/6/21	Gyulai (11), Székesfehérvár	65.20	65.45	67.71	x	x	65.44	65.950
75	67.65	4/16/22	MSR (62), Walnut, CA	65.72	66.30	67.65	x	65.92	66.96	66.510
76	67.64	8/4/17	WCh (16) - Q (64.50), London	61.83	67.64	-				64.735
77	67.64	6/22/21	Karlstad / Folksam GP, Karlstad	67.22	65.18	67.64	x	66.48	x	66.630
78	67.62	2/25/22	Diskustävling, Växjö	66.85	x	67.62	x	x	x	67.235
79	67.61	7/29/23	NC (128) (SWE Ch), Söderhamn	67.61	67.1	x	x	66.84	x	67.183
80	67.59	7/7/17	Club Ch Final, Borås	66.73	x	x	x	67.59	64.21	66.177
81	67.59	9/30/19	WCh (17), Doha	66.59	67.18	67.59	65.83	x	67.05	66.848
82	67.57	6/30/22	Bauhaus (56)/DL, Stockholm	x	63.90	x	65.03	67.57	66.16	65.665
83	67.57	7/2/23	Bauhaus (57)/DL, Stockholm	x	67.57	x	x	x	x	67.570
84	67.39	6/16/18	Bottnarydskastet, Bottnaryd	66.62	x	67.39	x	65.73	65.11	66.213
85	67.37	9/3/17	SWE v FIN, Stockholm	67.37	61.68	x	62.44	x	x	63.830
86	67.36	9/17/23	Prefontaine/DL, Eugene, OR	64.59	67.13	67.36	x	x	65.62	66.175
87	67.31	8/19/20	Gyulai (10), Székesfehérvár	66.52	65.17	x	67.31	66.67	x	66.418
88	67.30	8/5/23	Folksam GP, Malmö	67.3	x	x	65.89	x	66.13	66.440
89	67.28	9/6/20	Skolimowska (11), Chorzów	66.54	x	67.01	x	66.55	67.28	66.845
90	67.26	7/25/17	Karlstad / Folksam GP, Karlstad	64.11	66.07	65.47	65.35	58.64	67.26	64.483
91	67.25	6/24/23	ETC, Chorzów	67.25	x	x	x	x	x	67.250
92	67.24	9/4/23	Galà dei Castelli, Bellinzona	63.97	67.24	63.02	62.72	62.17	x	63.824
93	67.16	6/5/22	Mohammed VI/DL, ar-Rabāṭ	64.35	67.16	66.94	66.26	66.58	62.53	65.637
94	67.14	5/5/23	Diamond/DL, Doha	64.31	x	67.14	64.32	63.97	65.85	65.118

Table 15 (continued from previous page)

#	Mark	Date	Competition	Rnd 1	Rnd 2	Rnd 3	Rnd 4	Rnd 5	Rnd 6	series avg
			Daniel Ståhl All Time Performances as of 31.10.2023							
95	67.10	7/19/22	WCh (18), Eugene, OR	66.59	65.99	x	65.39	67.10	66.86	66.386
96	67.07	8/7/18	ECh (24) - Q (64.00), Berlin	67.07	-	-				67.070
97	67.04	6/7/18	Bislett/DL, Oslo	x	66.55	x	x	60.30	67.04	64.630
98	67.04	8/28/21	NC (126) (SWE Ch), Borås	64.53	66.79	67.04	66.09	x	63.80	65.650
99	67.03	7/23/23	DL/London Athletics Meet , London	x	64.89	x	67.03	x	x	65.960
100	67.01	8/8/22	Gyulai (12), Székesfehérvár	66.55	66.74	66.84	67.01	x	66.32	66.692
101	66.92	7/18/16	Gyulai (6), Székesfehérvár	63.13	66.28	65.27	x	66.92	66.34	65.588
102	66.90	2/11/17	FIN v 3-Nat, Tampere	x	x	x	57.89	66.90	x	62.395
103	66.89	5/3/14	Steve Scott Inv (20), Irvine, CA	63.48	66.89	x	x	59.54	61.00	62.728
104	66.89	8/31/23	Tallinn 2023, Tallinn	63.05	64.5	66.89	65.46	64.24	65.27	64.902
105	66.81	3/10/18	EP-w (18), Leiria	66.81	64.96	x	x	60.63	x	64.133
106	66.81	6/2/21	Göteborg / Folksam GP, Göteborg	x	66.81	x	x	x	x	66.810
107	66.75	7/3/22	Karlstad / Folksam GP, Karlstad	66.75	x	x	65.29	x	x	66.020
108	66.74	4/17/16	Spring Fling, Salinas, CA	?	?	66.74				66.740
109	66.74	8/31/18	VD (42)/DL, Bruxelles	65.59	64.63	x	65.86	66.74	63.35	65.234
110	66.73	7/9/17	Anniversary Games/DL, London	65.63	63.59	66.23	x	65.19	66.73	65.474
111	66.65	5/26/18	Werfertage (44), Halle (Saale)	x	x	63.01	x	62.49	66.65	64.050
112	66.55	7/4/20	Hässelby	x	66.45	66.55	66.42	x	x	66.473
113	66.49	9/9/21	Weltklasse/DL, Zürich	66.49	x	x	x	65.64	x	66.065
114	66.44	9/2/23	SWE v FIN, Stockholm	x	x	65.35	x	66.44	66.4	66.063
115	66.42	4/23/16	Triton Inv, La Jolla, CA	64.93	66.42	x	x	x	65.20	65.517
116	66.42	9/8/20	Golden Spike (59), Ostrava	63.90	66.01	66.42	x	x	66.00	65.583
117	66.41	6/25/17	ETC-1, Vaasa	x	66.41	x	65.63			66.020
118	66.39	8/17/22	ECh (25) - Q (66.00), München	66.39	-	-				66.390
119	66.39	8/19/22	ECh (25), München	66.39	65.80	64.76	63.42	65.94	66.00	65.385
120	66.26	6/18/22	Motonet GP, Kuortane	x	66.26	x	65.43	64.29	x	65.327
121	66.25	8/19/23	WCh (19) - Q (66.50), Budapest	64.58	66.25	64.99				65.273
122	66.17	6/28/18	Sollentuna / Folksam GP, Sollentuna	66.17	x	65.20	65.23	64.11	63.85	64.912
123	66.16	6/10/18	Bauhaus (52)/DL, Stockholm	66.16	64.46	x	x	x	x	65.310
124	66.12	7/30/21	Oly G - Q (66.00), Tōkyō	66.12	-	-				66.120
125	66.00	9/17/18	Castorama, Sätra	64.16	x	66.00	65.38			65.180
126	65.97	5/21/22	British GP/DL, Birmingham	65.86	65.97	x	x	65.52	x	65.783
127	65.95	3/12/22	EP-w (21), Leiria	61.90	x	65.95	x	64.12	x	63.990
128	65.95	7/17/22	WCh (18) - Q (66.00), Eugene, OR	x	65.95	x				65.950
129	65.92	6/11/20	Impossible Games, Oslo	x	x	64.92	x	65.92	x	65.420
130	65.89	9/13/20	ISTAF (79), Berlin	x	65.89	x	x	65.88	x	65.885
131	65.87	6/9/22	Golden Gala (42)/DL, Roma	65.68	63.85	65.87	x	x	65.133
132	65.78	7/7/16	ECh (23) - Q (64.00), Amsterdam	x	x	65.78				65.780
133	65.78	9/9/16	VD (40)/DL, Bruxelles	x	64.53	65.78	62.73	x	64.01	64.263
134	65.64	7/20/17	indoor, Växjö	62.53	x	65.36	x	65.64	64.42	64.488
135	65.46	9/3/16	FIN v SWE, Tampere	65.46	64.15	60.19	65.00	x	64.74	63.908
136	65.34	9/3/22	FIN v SWE, Helsinki	64.90	64.94	65.34	x	x	x	65.060
137	65.22	8/7/23	Victor Svanesohn Memorial , Helsingborg	x	x	x	65.22	x	x	65.220
138	65.16	9/8/22	Weltklasse/DL, Zürich	62.88	x	x	x	65.16	61.47	63.170
139	64.98	4/14/18	Triton Inv, La Jolla, CA	62.69	64.06	64.98	x	62.44	64.94	63.822
140	64.93	9/11/22	Hanžeković (72), Zagreb	x	64.93	x	x	x	x	64.930
141	64.92	6/27/20	Bottnarydskastet, Bottnaryd	64.92	62.65	63.86	64.05	x	63.18	63.732

Table 15 (continued from previous page)

#	Mark	Date	Competition	Rnd 1	Rnd 2	Rnd 3	Rnd 4	Rnd 5	Rnd 6	series avg
			Daniel Ståhl All Time Performances as of 31.10.2023							
142	64.91	9/13/18	GK viimane vaatus, Tallinn	x	64.91	63.14	64.84			64.297
143	64.84	5/31/18	Golden Gala (38)/DL, Roma	62.31	64.56	64.51	63.80	64.10	64.84	64.020
144	64.84	9/8/18	Continental Cup, Ostrava	64.84	x	x				64.840
145	64.77	7/9/16	ECh (23), Amsterdam	62.17	64.04	x	x	62.53	64.77	63.378
146	64.76	8/21/16	Folksam Chall, Helsingborg	59.84	62.64	62.59	60.32	x	64.76	62.030
147	64.73	8/29/15	WCh (15), Beijing	61.74	60.42	64.42	64.73	x	x	62.828
148	64.72	4/30/16	Steve Scott Inv (22), Irvine, CA	x	63.21	x	63.52	64.72	x	63.817
149	64.67	7/28/23	NC (128) (SWE Ch) - Q, Söderhamn	64.67	-	-				64.670
150	64.60	7/3/14	Athletissima/DL, Lausanne	60.66	63.55	60.73	x	64.60	60.62	62.032
151	64.46	7/2/18	Gyulai (8), Székesfehérvár	64.46	63.89	x	63.96	x	60.87	63.295
152	64.44	6/11/17	FBK-Games (35), Hengelo	x	63.74	x	64.44	x	63.58	63.920
153	64.35	4/21/18	Beach Inv, Long Beach, CA	63.60	61.68	63.15	x	x	64.35	63.195
154	64.30	4/24/14	HP/OTC Series I, Chula Vista, CA	x	64.30	61.66	58.98	58.00	62.10	61.008
155	64.24	7/27/16	Karlstad / Folksam GP, Karlstad	61.09	x	x	61.59	x	64.24	62.307
156	64.18	9/1/17	VD (41)/DL, Bruxelles	x	64.18	x	x	60.96	x	62.570
157	64.14	5/13/17	Diamond/DL, Shanghai	61.03	63.87	64.14	x	63.76	60.48	62.656
158	64.06	5/6/16	Diamond/DL, Doha	x	64.06	x				64.060
159	63.87	4/29/17	Steve Scott Inv (23), Irvine, CA	62.49	63.87	61.00	63.48	61.89	60.08	62.135
160	63.69	8/2/14	NC (119), Umeå	61.64	x	57.06	x	63.69	x	60.797
161	63.68	6/13/16	Sule (52), Tartu	x	62.24	x	x	63.05	63.68	62.990
162	63.61	7/27/14	Nordic Ch-j-22, København	x	62.03	59.64	60.25	63.61	x	61.383
163	63.47	6/16/16	Bauhaus (50), Stockholm	x	x	x	59.05	63.47	x	61.260
164	63.42	6/28/16	Sollentuna / Folksam GP, Sollentuna	63.42	x	59.12	x	x	x	61.270
165	63.38	7/1/15	Club Ch, Sundsvall	59.26	61.04	63.38	57.10	58.00	62.18	60.160
166	63.25	6/2/16	Golden Gala (36)/DL, Roma	62.11	63.25	60.46				61.940
167	63.20	8/10/15	Göteborg	x	x	60.19	x	x	63.20	61.695
168	63.16	4/28/18	Steve Scott Inv (24), Irvine, CA	x	x	63.16	x	62.56	x	62.860
169	63.09	4/26/14	Triton Inv, La Jolla, CA	63.09	54.91	57.50	55.53	x	x	57.758
170	63.03	7/30/15	Bauhaus (49)/DL, Stockholm	61.25	x	x	x	60.75	63.03	61.677
171	63.02	6/28/14	Bottnarydskastet, Bottnaryd	x	x	60.73	59.63	63.02	58.69	60.518
172	62.93	6/25/15	Sollentuna / Folksam GP, Sollentuna	x	60.16	x	x	x	62.93	61.545
173	62.87	7/15/16	Herculis/DL, Monaco	61.96	62.20	x	x	x	62.87	62.343
174	62.86	6/21/16	Folksam Chall, Umeå	62.61	x	x	x	x	62.86	62.735
175	62.85	6/27/15	Bottnarydskastet, Bottnaryd	x	59.57	x	62.85	x	x	61.210
176	62.76	7/19/15	Kalam, Viljandi	60.56	58.58	x	62.76	61.86	x	60.940
177	62.66	8/27/15	WCh (15) - Q (65.00), Beijing	62.66	61.22	62.06				61.980
178	62.62	6/12/14	M. Iberoamericano, Huelva	61.77	x	60.98	62.11	62.62	60.12	61.520
179	62.60	5/24/14	Grote Prijs, Lokeren	55.53	60.78	x	62.60	60.62	55.62	59.030
180	62.31	6/30/14	Göteborg	60.30	60.50	x	x	62.31		61.037
181	62.26	8/12/16	Oly G - Q (65.50), Rio de Janeiro	60.78	x	62.26				61.520
182	62.26	9/9/17	Castorama, Karlstad							
183	62.21	9/12/15	SWE v FIN, Stockholm	61.86	59.34	x	x	61.64	62.21	61.263
184	62.16	8/25/12	NC (117), Stockholm	61.11	x	62.16	61.38	x	61.03	61.420
185	62.05	6/5/14	Golden Gala (34)/DL, Roma	57.29	62.05	58.64	60.18	60.73	x	59.778
186	61.93	6/5/16	British GP/DL, Birmingham	60.80	x	61.93				61.365
187	61.80	9/14/16	Castorama, Sätra	61.80	x	x	p?			61.800
188	61.77	8/30/14	FIN v SWE, Helsinki	x	60.36	61.77	58.63	60.26	59.16	60.036

Table 15 (continued from previous page)

#	Mark	Date	Competition	Rnd 1	Rnd 2	Rnd 3	Rnd 4	Rnd 5	Rnd 6	series avg
			Daniel Ståhl All Time Performances as of 31.10.2023							
189	61.60	7/18/14	Herculis/DL, Monaco	61.60	61.42	x	x	x	61.37	61.463
190	61.51	3/11/17	EP-w (17), Las Palmas, G C	x	x	x	61.51	x	x	61.510
191	61.42	7/22/12	Nordic/Baltic Ch-j-22, Jessheim	58.20	61.42	60.94	x	60.89	x	60.363
192	61.38	8/11/19	ETC, Bydgoszcz	x	61.38	x	x			61.380
193	61.29	7/13/13	EJ-22 (9), Tampere	x	59.51	58.93	x	61.29	58.85	59.645
194	61.23	6/9/15	Sule (51), Tartu	x	61.23	x	x	x	x	61.230
195	61.12	8/16/15	Folksam Chall, Umeå	58.58	x	x	59.91	61.12	x	59.870
196	61.09	2/6/16	Botnia Games, Mustasaari	60.32	61.09	59.59	59.93	x	57.12	59.610
197	61.09	5/22/16	Mohammed VI/DL, ar-Rabāṭ	61.09	x	x				61.090
198	60.96	8/24/14	British GP/DL, Birmingham	59.56	x	x	x	x	60.96	60.260
199	60.77	7/14/15	Spitzen, Luzern	60.07	x	x	60.77	59.50	59.87	60.053
200	60.74	5/28/13	Sule (49), Tartu	54.66	59.04	x	x	56.03	60.74	57.618
201	60.68	5/10/14	København	x	60.68	x	55.13	x	54.96	56.923
202	60.60	7/5/14	Club Ch, Borås	x	58.35	x	60.60			59.475
203	60.55	6/14/15	EAF (15), Bydgoszcz	60.55	59.64	x	x	x	x	60.095
204	60.48	8/14/15	Folksam Chall, Göteborg	x	x	x	60.48	59.44	x	59.960
205	60.47	8/18/13	Folksam Chall, Umeå							
206	60.46	6/30/18	M. de Paris/DL, Charléty, Paris	x	60.46	x				60.460
207	60.37	6/7/15	Folksam Chall, Uppsala	x	x	x	x	55.96	60.37	58.165
208	60.28	6/26/14	Sollentuna / Folksam GP, Sollentuna	59.07	60.28	x	58.44	59.84	x	59.408
209	60.26	7/11/15	Meeting Madrid (33), Madrid	x	58.42	58.90	x	60.26	59.56	59.285
210	60.25	9/13/12	ERGO Mängud, Kose	56.02	60.25	x	x	57.14	58.05	57.865
211	60.20	8/8/15	NC (120) (SWE Ch), Söderhamn	59.39	x	60.20	x	x	x	59.795
212	60.09	2/8/14	FIN v 3-Nat, Tampere	57.62	58.48	57.65	60.09	x	54.77	57.722
213	59.98	8/4/12	Gurkspelen, Västerås							
214	59.83	7/7/13	Öresundsspelen, Helsingborg							
215	59.70	9/4/12	Hanžeković (62), Zagreb	59.70	x	59.18	x	x	57.78	58.887
216	59.59	7/17/13	Spitzen, Luzern	57.95	59.59	x	x	x	x	58.770
217	59.50	7/31/13	Night of Athletics, Göteborg							
218	59.34	5/18/14	Werfertage (40)-j-22, Halle (Saale)	57.13	x	59.25	x	x	59.34	58.573
219	59.30	8/11/13	NC-j-22, Växjö							
220	59.29	9/2/12	SWE v FIN, Göteborg	58.86	59.29	x	55.24	x	55.22	57.153
221	59.07	8/31/13	NC (118), Borås	58.88	58.21	59.07	x	x	x	58.720
222	59.05	9/5/15	Göteborg / Folksam GP, Göteborg	59.05	x	x	x	x	x	59.050
223	59.01	8/12/14	ECh (22) - Q (64.00), Zürich	x	56.51	59.01				57.760
224	58.94	8/3/15	Kasttävling, Helsingborg	58.59	58.94	55.97	56.45	x	58.15	57.620
225	58.74	8/3/13	Folksam Chall, Mölndal	x	55.99	58.74	56.24	x	58.12	57.273
226	58.67	6/3/12	Heitjate sv II etapp, Tallinn	54.80	x	57.02	58.67	x	x	56.830
227	58.65	9/16/12	Castorama, Sätra							
228	58.61	6/27/13	Sollentuna / Folksam GP, Sollentuna	58.61	x	x	55.36	54.96	x	56.310
229	58.49	3/22/14	Wexiö Indoor Throws, Växjö	x	58.49	x	56.77	56.20	55.55	56.753
230	58.46	9/22/13	Castorama, Sätra							
231	58.41	6/16/12	Bottnarydskastet cB, Bottnaryd	55.51	56.09	55.91	52.59	x	58.41	55.702
232	58.30	9/7/13	SWE v FIN, Stockholm	58.30	57.65	x	x	56.52	x	57.490
233	58.19	7/2/13	Växjö							
234	57.93	6/10/12	Helsingborg Throws-j-22, Helsingborg							
235	57.88	6/17/12	Helsingborg Throws-j-22, Helsingborg							

Table 15 (continued from previous page)

#	Mark	Date	Competition	Rnd 1	Rnd 2	Rnd 3	Rnd 4	Rnd 5	Rnd 6	series avg
			Daniel Ståhl All Time Performances as of 31.10.2023							
236	57.87	6/28/15	Kasttävling, Helsingborg							
237	57.83	6/9/12	Helsingborg Throws-j-22, Helsingborg							
238	57.80	9/2/14	Castorama, Växjö							
239	57.77	7/12/12	Sätra							
240	57.77	6/14/13	Göteborg							
241	57.70	3/15/14	EP-w (14)-j-22, Leiria	x	56.40	57.70	56.66	x	57.61	57.093
242	57.45	3/17/12	EP-w (12)-j-22, Bar	53.45	x	54.30	57.22	x	57.45	55.605
243	57.44	7/11/13	EJ-22 (9) - Q (59.50), Tampere	56.96	57.44	56.10				56.833
244	57.44	7/28/13	HAIS-Spelen, Hässleholm	x	57.44	x	x	56.63	56.46	56.843
245	57.32	7/5/12	Sollentuna / Folksam GP, Sollentuna	x	57.32	57.32				57.320
246	57.24	6/22/14	ETC, Braunschweig	x	57.24	57.12				57.180
247	57.14	6/30/12	Uppsala							
248	56.86	1/10/13	Cougar Inv, Provo, UT	56.16	x	56.86	x	x	x	56.510
249	56.84	2/13/16	ISTAF Indoor (3), Berlin	x	x	x	x	x	56.84	56.840
250	56.82	7/3/12	BIGBANK, Viljandi	53.40	56.08	56.82				55.433
251	56.67	3/16/13	EP-w (13)-j-22, Castellón	x	x	x	56.67	55.62	x	56.145
252	56.39	6/29/12	Bottnarydskastet, Bottnaryd	x	x	56.39	55.36	x	54.61	55.453
253	56.23	8/7/12	Stockholm							
254	56.20	4/26/12	Triton Inv Elite, La Jolla, CA	55.45	56.20	56.07				55.907
255	56.15	7/15/12	Sätra							
256	56.11	4/27/13	Triton Inv, La Jolla, CA							
257	55.75	3/10/12	Wexiö Ind Throws-j-22, Växjö	53.50	x	54.39	55.75	53.93	54.52	54.418
258	55.65	5/5/12	Oxy Inv, Eagle Rock, CA	52.65	53.92	55.46	55.65			54.420
259	55.60	8/13/11	NC (116), Gävle							
260	55.13	5/3/12	OTC Pre-Oly II, Chula Vista, CA	55.13	54.40	x	52.73	55.07	x	54.333
261	54.92	8/8/11	Kasttävling, Helsingborg	x	50.44	54.92	52.66	x	x	52.673
262	54.91	5/20/13	Hulst							
263	54.66	4/25/13	Triton Inv Elite, La Jolla, CA	54.66	x	x				54.660
264	54.63	5/19/13	Grote Prijs, Lokeren	x	x	54.63	54.37	x	x	54.500
265	54.36	4/28/12	Triton Inv Open, La Jolla, CA							
266	54.36	6/13/13	Bislett/DL, Oslo	54.36	x	x				54.360
267	54.09	5/20/12	Werfertage (38)-j-22, Halle (Saale)	53.80	54.09	x	53.84	53.97	x	53.925
268	54.00	5/26/12	Mästarmöte i kast, Nyköping	54.00	x	x	x	53.44	x	53.720
269	53.53	4/20/13	Soka Peace Inv, Aliso Viejo, CA							
270	53.00	9/24/11	Kasttävling, Helsingborg	51.64	53.00	x	51.92	52.53	x	52.273
271	52.76	5/29/12	Sule (48), Tartu	51.58	52.76	x				52.170
272	52.38	5/12/12	Vårkastet, Bålsta	x	x	52.38	x	51.19	x	51.785
273	50.32	8/21/10	NC (115), Falun							
274	50.18	4/16/11	Mark Faldmo Inv, Logan, UT							
275	49.77	4/23/11	Robison Inv, Provo, UT	x	x	x	x	x	49.77	49.770
276	0	8/22/13	DN Galan (47)/DL, Stockholm	x	x	x				
277	0	6/21/15	ETC, Cheboksary	x	x	x				
278	0	9/6/15	ISTAF (74), Berlin	x	x	x				
279	0	8/18/18	Göteborg / Folksam GP, Göteborg	x	x	x	x	x	x	
280	0	6/11/19	PNG (57), Turku	x	x	x				
281	0	6/14/20	Södertälje	x	x	x	x	x	x	
282	0	3/7/21	Diskustävling, Växjö	x	x	x	x	x	x	

Table 16

#	Mark	Name	Comp	Date	1	2	3	4	5	6	series avg
			All Time Best Performances with Series Average (as of 31.10.2023)								
1	74.08	Jürgen Schult	EC Q Meet (WR), Neubrandenburg	6/6/1986	67.20	x	x	74.08	x	p	70.640
2	73.88	Virgilijus Alekna	NC (77), Kaunas	8/3/2000	70.22	72.35	69.26	73.88	x	x	71.428
3	73.38	Gerd Kanter	Helsingborg	9/4/2006	69.46	72.30	70.43	73.38	70.51	65.88	70.327
4	72.02	Gerd Kanter	comp 1, Salinas, CA	5/3/2007	70.52	68.02	x	x	72.02	68.50	69.765
5	71.88	Gerd Kanter	comp A, Salinas, CA	5/8/2008	~67.5	~68	~69	~68.5	x	71.88	71.880
6	71.86	Yuriy Dumchev	Moscow Ch (WR), Moskva	5/29/1983	x	x	64.58	66.22	70.60	71.86	68.315
7	71.86	Daniel Ståhl	Bottnarydskastet, Bottnaryd	6/29/2019	68.76	68.83	69.71	x	71.86	x	69.790
8	71.86	Kristjan Čeh	Heino Lipp (15), Jõhvi	6/16/2023	68.93	x	67.92	71.70	71.19	71.86	70.320
9	71.84	Piotr Małachowski	FBK-Games (31), Hengelo	6/8/2013	65.53	x	x	67.73	71.84	x	68.367
10	71.70	Róbert Fazekas	MAL, Szombathely	7/14/2002	62.82	x	69.96	x	71.70	x	68.160
11	71.64	Gerd Kanter	BIGBANK, Kohila	6/25/2009	x	69.93	x	71.64	68.03	70.92	70.130
12	71.56	Virgilijus Alekna	Kaunas 2007, Kaunas	7/25/2007	65.29	67.65	67.62	67.37	x	71.56	67.898
13	71.50	Lars Riedel	WLV Diskus-Cup, Wiesbaden	5/3/1997	64.10	66.94	65.26	70.84	68.94	71.50	67.930
14	71.47	Daniel Ståhl	Club Ch, Uppsala	6/21/2022	67.05	x	71.47	69.51	x	68.15	69.045
15	71.46	Daniel Ståhl	WCh (19), Budapest	8/21/2023	63.01	66.58	x	69.37	67.56	71.46	67.596
16	71.45	Gerd Kanter	Throws II, Chula Vista, CA	4/29/2010	67.98	61.68	65.81	67.15	71.45	67.06	66.855
17	71.45	Daniel Ståhl	Heino Lipp (15), Jõhvi	6/16/2023	66.28	x	x	67.20	x	71.45	68.310
18	71.40	Daniel Ståhl	Bottnarydskastet, Bottnaryd	7/10/2021	70.27	71.40	x	64.67	x	x	68.780
19	71.37	Daniel Ståhl	Sollentuna / Folksam GP, Sollentuna	8/10/2020	68.38	x	71.37	x	x	x	69.875
20	71.32	Ben Plucknett	Prefontaine, Eugene, Oregon	6/4/1983	67.32	62.14	x	69.50	71.08	71.32	68.272
21	71.29	Daniel Ståhl	Sollentuna / Folksam GP, Sollentuna	6/29/2017	68.88	x	71.29	x	x	62.83	67.667
22	71.27	Kristjan Čeh	British GP/DL, Birmingham	5/21/2022	67.77	69.10	71.27	63.11	69.33	65.28	67.643
23	71.26	John Powell	TAC (96), San José, CA	6/9/1984	67.72	67.18	67.04	69.82	71.26	x	68.604
24	71.26	Rickard Bruch	Malmö	11/15/1984	66.28	66.32	67.41	68.48	71.26	x	67.950
25	71.26	Imrich Bugár	Jenner Classic, San José, CA	5/25/1985	71.26	65.68	68.88	67.88	x	x	68.425
26	71.25	Róbert Fazekas	World Cup (9), Madrid	9/21/2002	65.41	71.25	69.77	x			68.810
27	71.25	Virgilijus Alekna	Daněk Memorial (10), Turnov	5/20/2008	67.93	x	67.37	67.86	69.32	71.25	68.746
28	71.23	Kristjan Čeh	Gyulai (12), Székesfehérvár	8/8/2022	71.23	70.35	68.00	65.39	x	x	68.743
29	71.17	Art Burns	All Comers, San José, CA	7/19/1983	x	53.19	71.17	x	61.29	x	61.883
30	71.16	Wolfgang Schmidt	EM Test (WR), Berlin	8/9/1978	68.14	71.16	67.72	67.16	65.78	68.34	68.050
31	71.14	Ben Plucknett	Kinney Inv, Berkeley, CA	6/12/1983	68.04	71.14	x	x	69.32	64.92	68.355
32	71.14	Anthony Washington	Hartnell, Salinas, CA	5/22/1996	67.66	x	x	71.14	x	65.52	68.107
33	71.13	Kristjan Čeh	WCh (18), Eugene, Oregon	7/19/2022	65.27	69.02	71.13	68.95	70.51	67.57	68.742
34	71.12	Virgilijus Alekna	Weltklasse, Zürich	8/11/2000	70.26	68.55	68.68	70.42	70.60	71.12	69.938
35	71.08	Virgilijus Alekna	Vardinoyiánnia (22), Réthymno	7/21/2006	68.55	70.12	67.80	66.72	66.80	71.08	68.512
36	71.06	Luis Mariano Delís	Barrientos (33), La Habana	5/21/1983	x	68.84	69.52	x	71.06	68.74	69.540
37	71.06	Lars Riedel	Weltklasse, Zürich	8/14/1996	66.98	68.64	69.32	69.26	70.38	71.06	69.273
38	71.00	Rickard Bruch	Malmö	10/14/1984	69.82	71.00	68.64	69.68	70.18	65.02	69.057
39	71.00	Mykolas Alekna	Cal v Stanford, Berkeley, CA	4/29/2023	63.29	67.25	71.00	x	66.21	p	66.938
40	70.99	Virgilijus Alekna	Engen, Stellenbosch	3/30/2001	70.59	66.11	x	x	70.99	x	69.230
41	70.98	Mac Wilkins	WG (14), Helsinki	7/9/1980	70.98	x	67.24	70.20	65.14	68.32	68.376
42	70.98	Art Burns	Prefontaine, Eugene, Oregon	7/21/1984	62.52	65.94	67.22	68.48	67.08	70.98	67.037
43	70.97	Virgilijus Alekna	Vardinoyiánnia (20), Réthymno	6/23/2004	68.61	69.08	70.02	67.85	70.97	68.76	69.215
44	70.93	Gerd Kanter	Helsingborg	6/28/2007	70.93	68.79	x	x	70.73	70.14	70.148
45	70.93	Daniel Ståhl	Sollentuna / Folksam GP, Sollentuna	6/11/2023	68.24	67.09	x	68.16	70.93	x	68.605
46	70.92	Wolfgang Schmidt	Norder Werferserie, Norden	9/9/1989	66.48	70.92	x	64.56	66.42	67.54	67.184
47	70.92	Gerd Kanter	Kaunas 2007, Kaunas	7/25/2007	66.79	x	66.62	69.92	x	70.92	68.563
48	70.89	Daniel Ståhl	Varberg / Folksam GP, Varberg	7/15/2019	67.99	68.79	70.78	70.36	70.89	70.37	69.863
49	70.89	Kristjan Čeh	Diamond/DL, Doha	5/5/2023	70.89	x	68.95	68.46	70.70	x	69.750
50	70.86	Mac Wilkins	San José Inv (WR), San José, CA	5/1/1976	69.80	70.24	70.86	66.98	68.08	66.58	68.757

Table 16 (continued from previous page)

	**All Time Best Performances with Series Average (as of 31.10.2023)**

#	Mark	Name	Comp	Date	1	2	3	4	5	6	series avg
51	70.86	Virgilijus Alekna	Vardinoyiánnia (24), Réthymno	7/14/2008	67.95	70.55	x	70.86	70.76	x	70.030
52	70.84	Gerd Kanter	WRC, Chula Vista, CA	4/28/2009	x	70.84	x	69.05	x	x	69.945
53	70.83	Róbert Fazekas	Vardinoyiánnia (20), Réthymno	6/23/2004	66.48	x	70.83	x	67.65	69.87	68.708
54	70.82	Aleksander Tammert	Mean Green, Denton, Texas	4/15/2006	64.76	68.04	x	66.28	65.62	70.82	67.104
55	70.81	Ben Plucknett	Hartnell, Salinas, CA	6/1/1983	64.56	68.58	70.81	69.44	x	69.47	68.572
56	70.78	Róbert Fazekas	Budapest	5/10/2003	64.77	68.56	70.78	68.78	69.34	x	68.446
57	70.78	Fedrick Dacres	Mohammed VI/DL, ar-Rabāṭ	6/16/2019	67.09	68.71	70.78	69.50	68.83	x	68.982
58	70.72	Imrich Bugár	AUT v HUN v TCH, Schwechat	6/18/1983	67.46	69.30	68.98	67.98	70.72	66.38	68.470
59	70.72	Kristjan Čeh	Golden Gala (42)/DL, Roma	6/9/2022	66.48	x	68.76	69.06	69.71	70.72	68.946
60	70.68	Lukas Weißhaidinger	Helvetia Discuswurf, Schwechat	5/19/2023	68.36	70.68	x	x	x	x	69.520
61	70.67	Virgilijus Alekna	Meeting Madrid (23), Madrid	7/16/2005	66.49	68.60	x	69.97	70.67	x	68.933
62	70.66	Mac Wilkins	AAU (91), Walnut, CA	6/16/1979	62.98	70.66	x	67.20	66.66	66.88	66.876
63	70.66	Robert Harting	Daněk Memorial (13), Turnov	5/22/2012	69.18	x	70.66	x	x	66.33	68.723
64	70.62	Daniel Ståhl	PNG (60), Turku	6/14/2022	70.62	x	x	67.75	64.55	x	67.640
65	70.61	Virgilijus Alekna	Tammert, Tallinn	9/16/2005	66.03	68.35	65.21	68.97	68.10	70.61	67.878
66	70.60	Lars Riedel	ISTAF (55), Berlin	8/30/1996	67.58	70.60	68.24	66.38	70.38	x	68.636
67	70.58	Luis Mariano Delís	Hartnell, Salinas, CA	5/19/1982	x	67.49	x	65.45	70.00	70.58	68.380
68	70.58	Virgilijus Alekna	Vardinoyiánnia (21), Réthymno	7/10/2005	67.80	x	67.84	69.86	70.58	67.25	68.666
69	70.56	Daniel Ståhl	Diamond/DL, Doha	5/3/2019	69.63	70.49	70.56	69.54	69.50	70.32	70.007
70	70.55	Daniel Ståhl	Motonet GP, Kuortane	6/26/2021	63.61	x	69.99	70.21	x	70.55	68.590
71	70.54	Dmitriy Shevchenko	Kuban, Krasnodar	5/7/2002	68.93	70.54	x	p	67.44	p	68.970
72	70.54	Kristjan Čeh	NC, Velenje	7/9/2023	x	65.70	68.29	70.54	62.58	64.17	66.256
73	70.53	Virgilijus Alekna	Athletissima, Lausanne	7/5/2005	67.92	67.79	68.69	70.53	x	x	68.733
74	70.51	Virgilijus Alekna	Bislett, Oslo	6/15/2007	67.95	70.51	66.94	67.16	x	x	68.140
75	70.48	Mac Wilkins	San José Inv, San José, CA	4/29/1978	70.48	70.10	x	x	x	x	70.290
76	70.48	Mac Wilkins	Prefontaine, Eugene, Oregon	5/31/1978	66.24	67.70	69.02	70.48	69.40	70.42	68.877
77	70.48	Rickard Bruch	Malmö	9/12/1984	64.56	65.06	67.28	70.48	68.74	67.62	67.290
78	70.46	Jürgen Schult	Berlin	9/13/1988	67.28	70.46	69.76	68.22	69.86	p	69.116
79	70.44	Mac Wilkins	TAC (96), San José, CA	6/9/1984	70.44	x	67.38	67.74	x	68.46	68.505
80	70.43	Virgilijus Alekna	Tsiklitiria, Athína	7/2/2007	x	66.44	67.69	67.97	x	70.43	68.133
81	70.42	Simon Pettersson	NC (127) (SWE Ch), Norrköping	8/6/2022	69.84	67.67	x	66.79	70.42	x	68.680
82	70.40	Mykolas Alekna	Pac-12, Walnut, CA	5/14/2023	69.03	x	68.11	70.40	67.39	69.47	68.880
83	70.39	Virgilijus Alekna	Sule (36), Tartu	6/11/2000	68.34	70.06	68.99	70.39	68.30	x	69.216
84	70.39	Alex Rose	Oklahoma Throws #3, Ramona, OK	4/16/2023	67.92	64.38	x	65.80	70.39	61.66	66.030
85	70.38	Jay Silvester	Lancaster, CA	5/16/1971	70.38						70.380
86	70.38	Gerd Kanter	CV Throws, Chula Vista, CA	5/2/2008	69.54	68.32	x	66.95	65.26	70.38	68.090
87	70.38	Daniel Ståhl	PNG (61), Turku	6/13/2023	64.21	x	65.43	67.60	70.38	69.63	67.450
88	70.36	Mac Wilkins	S&W (42), Modesto, CA	5/14/1983	x	66.30	69.38	x	68.76	70.36	68.700
89	70.36	Gerd Kanter	Kópavogur	7/8/2007	63.68	63.96	65.61	69.96	70.36	67.91	66.913
90	70.35	Kristjan Čeh	Motonet GP, Kuortane	6/26/2021	x	67.81	70.35	x	68.54	70.22	69.230
91	70.32	Frantz Kruger	Salon-de-Provence	5/26/2002	59.17	68.73	66.32	67.64	x	70.32	66.436
92	70.32	Gerd Kanter	WRC, Helsingborg	9/6/2008	66.98	69.19	x	70.32	69.12	70.23	69.168
93	70.32	Kristjan Čeh	MohammedVI/DL, ar-Rabāṭ	5/28/2023	70.07	69.38	68.26	69.10	70.32	69.20	69.388
94	70.31	Robert Harting	Werfertage (38), Halle (Saale)	5/19/2012	x	66.41	70.31	x	x	x	68.360
95	70.30	Yuriy Dumchev	Bryansk	7/31/1988	67.60	67.80	70.30	68.50	68.68	68.60	68.580
96	70.29	Mauricio Ortega	Jornada Lançamentos, Vila Nova de Cerveira,	7/22/2020	x	59.49	61.65	70.29	x	x	63.810
97	70.29	Daniel Ståhl	NC (127) (SWE Ch), Norrköping	8/6/2022	68.67	68.37	68.97	66.54	70.29	69.07	68.652
98	70.28	Virgilijus Alekna	Klaipėda Ch, Klaipėda	6/23/2012	x	68.03	70.28	66.64	x	66.43	67.845
99	70.26	Imrich Bugár	ITA v TCH, Cagliari	9/8/1984	64.46	68.64	66.94	65.76	68.34	70.26	67.400
100	70.25	Daniel Ståhl	Helsingborg	6/21/2020	66.35	65.25	70.25	68.34	68.41	63.62	67.037

Table 17

Pos	Dist (M)	Athlete	DOB	Active
	**Men's Best Discus Throwers Using TOP-10 Throw Avg**
	as of 15.10.2023
1	71.380	Gerd Kanter, EST	06.05.1979	2006 - 2010
2	71.299	Virgilijus Alekna, LTU	13.02.1972	2000 - 2008
3	71.274	Daniel Ståhl, SWE	27.08.1992	2017 - 2023
4	70.833	Kristjan Čeh, SLO	17.02.1999	2021 - 2023
5	70.438	Mac Wilkins, USA	15.11.1950	1976 - 1984
6	70.258	Róbert Fazekas, HUN	18.08.1975	2002 - 2004
7	70.124	Imrich Bugár, CZE	14.04.1955	1983 - 1985
8	70.036	Lars Riedel, GER	28.06.1967	1996 - 2003
9	69.956	Luis Mariano Delís, CUB	06.12.1957	1982 - 1985
10	69.774	Jürgen Schult, GDR / GER	11.05.1960	1984 - 1992
11	69.635	Rickard Bruch, SWE	02.07.1946	1971 - 1984
12	69.614	Wolfgang Schmidt, GDR / FRG	16.01.1954	1978 - 1989
13	69.584	Robert Harting, GER	18.10.1984	2009 - 2013
14	69.546	Art Burns, USA	19.07.1954	1982 - 1986
15	69.505	Mykolas Alekna, LTU	18.09.2002	2022 - 2023
16	69.275	Piotr Małachowski, POL	07.06.1983	2008 - 2014
17	69.165	Andrius Gudžius, LTU	14.02.1991	2017 - 2023
18	69.136	Fedrick Dacres, JAM	28.02.1994	2017 - 2020
19	68.983	Lukas Weißhaidinger, AUT	20.02.1992	2018 - 2023
20	68.813	Ben Plucknett, USA	13.04.1954	1980 - 1983
21	68.795	Frantz Kruger, RSA / FIN	22.05.1975	2000 - 2007
22	68.754	John Powell, USA	25.06.1947	1974 - 1984
23	68.738	Anthony Washington, USA	16.01.1966	1996 - 1999
24	68.628	Zoltán Kővágó, HUN	10.04.1979	2004 - 2011
25	68.532	Knut Hjeltnes, NOR	08.12.1951	1979 - 1986
26	68.450	Ehsan Hadadi, IRI	21.01.1985	2007 - 2018
27	68.414	Yuriy Dumchev, RUS	05.08.1958	1980 - 1988
28	68.282	Juan Martínez Brito, CUB	17.05.1958	1983 - 1990
29	68.268	Romas Ubartas, LTU	26.05.1960	1986 - 1992
30	68.173	Mario Pestano, ESP	08.04.1978	2001 - 2011
31	68.122	Mike Buncic, USA	25.07.1962	1987 - 1993
32	68.071	Géjza Valent, CZE	03.10.1953	1982 - 1985
33	67.875	Simon Pettersson, SWE	03.01.1994	2020 - 2022
34	67.798	Aleksander Tammert, EST	02.02.1973	1999 - 2006
35	67.772	John Godina, USA	31.05.1972	1997 - 2001
36	67.687	Jarred Rome, USA	21.12.1976	2004 - 2011
37	67.660	Art Swarts, USA	14.02.1945	1977 - 1985
38	67.619	Ian Waltz, USA	15.04.1977	2005 - 2008
39	67.586	Alex Rose, SAM	17.11.1991	2021 - 2023
40	67.470	Georgiy Kolnootchenko, BLR	07.05.1959	1980 - 1986
41	67.463	Markku Tuokko, FIN	24.06.1951	1979 - 1981
42	67.362	Armin Lemme, GDR	28.10.1955	1981 - 1986

Table 17 (continued from previous page)

Men's Best Discus Throwers Using TOP-10 Throw Avg
as of 15.10.2023

Pos	Dist (M)	Athlete	DOB	Active
43	67.354	Stefan Fernholm, SWE	02.07.1959	1985 - 1990
44	67.337	Jay Silvester, USA	27.08.1937	1968 - 1973
45	67.274	Vaclovas Kidykas, LTU	17.10.1961	1985 - 1990
46	67.270	Yennifer Frank Casañas, CUB / ESP	18.10.1978	2006 - 2012
47	67.260	Erik de Bruin, NED	25.05.1963	1986 - 1993
48	67.255	Michael Möllenbeck, GER	12.12.1969	1996 - 2003
49	67.247	Traves Smikle, JAM	07.05.1992	2012 - 2023
50	67.236	Kenneth Stadel, USA	19.02.1952	1977 - 1982
51	67.207	Dmitriy Shevchenko, RUS	13.05.1968	1992 - 2002
52	67.182	Rolf Danneberg, FRG	01.03.1953	1984 - 1989
53	67.154	Christoph Harting, GER	04.10.1990	2015 - 2019
54	67.123	Matthew Denny, AUS	02.06.1996	2021 - 2023
55	67.121	Svein Inge Valvik, NOR	20.09.1956	1980 - 1987
56	67.087	Alfred "Al" Oerter, USA	19.09.1936	1979 - 1983
57	67.049	Martin Wierig, GER	10.06.1987	2011 - 2018
58	67.006	Uladzimir Dubrovchik, BLR	07.01.1972	1995 - 2000
59	66.981	John van Reenen, RSA	26.03.1947	1972 - 1976
60	66.966	Lawrence Okoye, GBR	06.10.1991	2011 - 2022
61	66.887	Philip Milanov, BEL	06.07.1991	2015 - 2023
62	66.858	Dmytro Kovtsun, UKR	29.09.1955	1980 - 1992
63	66.813	Rutger Smith, NED	09.07.1981	2007 - 2012
64	66.806	Jason Tunks, CAN	07.05.1975	1998 - 2006
65	66.798	Sam Mattis, USA	19.03.1994	2016 - 2023
66	66.781	Jason Young, USA	27.05.1981	2006 - 2011
67	66.774	Volodymyr Zinchenko, UKR	25.07.1959	1980 - 1988
68	66.768	Lois Maikel Martínez, CUB / ESP	03.06.1981	2005 - 2019
69	66.690	Alwin Wagner, FRG	11.08.1950	1977 - 1988
70	66.676	Vasiliy Kaptyukh, BLR	27.06.1967	1993 - 2003
71	66.666	Adam Setliff, USA	15.12.1969	1996 - 2001
72	66.592	Ludvík Daněk, CZE	06.01.1937	1969 - 1975
73	66.590	Wolfgang Warnemünde, GDR	08.05.1953	1980 - 1984
74	66.590	Daniel Jasinski, GER	05.08.1989	2014 - 2023
75	66.574	Attila Horváth, HUN	28.07.1967	1991 - 1998
76	66.526	Benn Harradine, AUS	14.10.1982	2008 - 2015
77	66.504	Erik Cadée, NED	15.02.1984	2010 - 2012
78	66.392	Andy Bloom, USA	11.08.1973	1997 - 2004
79	66.385	Roland Varga, HUN / CRO	22.10.1977	2001 - 2011
80	66.361	Mason Finley, USA	07.10.1990	2016 - 2021
81	66.318	Ihor Duginyets, UKR	20.05.1956	1980 - 1988
82	66.302	Mauricio Ortega, COL	04.08.1994	2016 - 2021
83	66.296	Iosif Nagy, ROU	20.11.1946	1979 - 1985
84	66.214	Reggie Jagers, USA	13.08.1994	2018 - 2021

Table 17 (continued from previous page)

Pos	Dist (M)	Athlete	DOB	Active
		**Men's Best Discus Throwers Using TOP-10 Throw Avg**		

Pos	Dist (M)	Athlete	DOB	Active
		Men's Best Discus Throwers Using TOP-10 Throw Avg		
		as of 15.10.2023		
85	66.178	Siegfried Pachale, GDR	24.10.1949	1973 - 1976
86	66.094	Velko Velev, BUL	04.01.1948	1975 - 1984
87	66.087	Pentti Kahma, FIN	03.12.1943	1973 - 1976
88	66.086	Marco Martino, ITA	21.02.1960	1984 - 1989
89	66.069	Robert Urbanek, POL	29.04.1987	2012 - 2020
90	65.982	Hilmar Hoßfeld, GDR	18.01.1954	1980 - 1984
91	65.970	Märt Israel, EST	23.09.1983	2007 - 2011
92	65.962	Nick Sweeney, IRL	26.03.1968	1994 - 1998
93	65.950	Julian Wruck, AUS	06.07.1991	2011 - 2014
94	65.949	Alin Alexandru Firfirica, ROU	03.11.1995	2018 - 2022
95	65.937	Casey Malone, USA	06.04.1977	2002 - 2010
96	65.842	Ion Zamfirache, ROU	23.08.1953	1982 - 1985
97	65.814	Marco Bucci, ITA	29.11.1960	1984 - 1985
98	65.814	Gábor Máté, HUN	09.02.1979	2000 - 2008
99	65.745	Kamy Keshmiri, USA	23.01.1969	1989 - 1991
100	65.724	Vésteinn Hafsteinsson, ISL	12.12.1960	1983 - 1994

Table 18

Pos	Dist (m)	Athlete	DOB	Active
	Men's Best Discus Throwers Using TOP-50 Throw Avg			
	as of 18.09.2023			
1	70.042	Virgilijus Alekna, LTU	13.02.1972	1998 - 2012
2	69.725	Daniel Ståhl, SWE	27.08.1992	2016 - 2023
3	69.648	Gerd Kanter, EST	06.05.1979	2004 - 2010
4	68.820	Mac Wilkins, USA	15.11.1950	1976 - 1988
5	68.806	Lars Riedel, GER	28.06.1967	1991 - 2006
6	68.761	Kristjan Čeh, SLO	17.02.1999	2020 - 2023
7	68.631	Luis Mariano Delís, CUB	06.12.1957	1980 - 1989
8	68.379	Robert Harting, GER	18.10.1984	2008 - 2016
9	68.296	Imrich Bugár, CZE	14.04.1955	1981 - 1987
10	68.104	Wolfgang Schmidt, GDR / FRG	16.01.1954	1976 - 1990
11	67.944	Piotr Małachowski, POL	07.06.1983	2008 - 2019
12	67.903	Andrius Gudžius, LTU	14.02.1991	2017 - 2023
13	67.795	Art Burns, USA	19.07.1954	1980 - 1987
14	67.760	Róbert Fazekas, HUN	18.08.1975	1998 - 2010
15	67.742	Jürgen Schult, GDR / GER	11.05.1960	1983 - 1999
16	67.635	Fedrick Dacres, JAM	28.02.1994	2014 - 2023
17	67.563	Rickard Bruch, SWE	02.07.1946	1969 - 1984
18	67.244	John Powell, USA	25.06.1947	1973 - 1987
19	67.130	Lukas Weißhaidinger, AUT	20.02.1992	2015 - 2023
20	67.023	Knut Hjeltnes, NOR	08.12.1951	1979 - 1987
21	66.890	Zoltán Kővágó, HUN	10.04.1979	2000 - 2017
22	66.839	Romas Ubartas, LTU	26.05.1960	1981 - 1992
23	66.788	Frantz Kruger, RSA / FIN	22.05.1975	1998 - 2008
24	66.712	Ehsan Hadadi, IRI	21.01.1985	2005 - 2019
25	66.673	Mario Pestano, ESP	08.04.1978	2001 - 2014
26	66.467	Géjza Valent, CZE	03.10.1953	1981 - 1988
27	66.442	Juan Martínez Brito, CUB	17.05.1958	1980 - 1990
28	66.437	Aleksander Tammert, EST	02.02.1973	1998 - 2012
29	66.357	Anthony Washington, USA	16.01.1966	1989 - 2000
30	66.206	Rolf Danneberg, FRG	01.03.1953	1984 - 1990
31	66.138	Simon Pettersson, SWE	03.01.1994	2017 - 2023
32	66.103	Mike Buncic, USA	25.07.1962	1984 - 1995
33	66.030	Yuriy Dumchev, RUS	05.08.1958	1980 - 1988
34	65.983	Yennifer Frank Casañas, CUB / ESP	18.10.1978	2003 - 2016
35	65.978	Michael Möllenbeck, GER	12.12.1969	1993 - 2007
36	65.836	Vaclovas Kidykas, LTU	17.10.1961	1985 - 1999
37	65.789	Jarred Rome, USA	21.12.1976	2001 - 2012
38	65.773	Martin Wierig, GER	10.06.1987	2010 - 2022
39	65.765	Ben Plucknett, USA	13.04.1954	1979 - 1983
40	65.738	Markku Tuokko, FIN	24.06.1951	1973 - 1982
41	65.698	John Godina, USA	31.05.1972	1995 - 2008
42	65.551	Ian Waltz, USA	15.04.1977	1998 - 2011
43	65.518	Alwin Wagner, FRG	11.08.1950	1977 - 1990

Table 18 (continued from previous page)

	Men's Best Discus Throwers Using TOP-50 Throw Avg			
	as of 18.09.2023			
Pos	Dist (m)	Athlete	DOB	Active
44	65.396	Stefan Fernholm, SWE	02.07.1959	1984 - 1996
45	65.392	Jason Tunks, CAN	07.05.1975	1997 - 2006
46	65.390	Art Swarts, USA	14.02.1945	1976 - 1986
47	65.377	Philip Milanov, BEL	06.07.1991	2014 - 2023
48	65.364	Erik de Bruin, NED	25.05.1963	1984 - 1993
49	65.318	Ludvík Daněk, CZE	06.01.1937	1964 - 1977
50	65.295	Traves Smikle, JAM	07.05.1992	2012 - 2023
51	65.262	Erik Cadée, NED	15.02.1984	2009 - 2017
52	65.233	Lawrence Okoye, GBR	06.10.1991	2011 - 2023
53	65.227	Jay Silvester, USA	27.08.1937	1965 - 1976
54	65.195	Kenneth Stadel, USA	19.02.1952	1973 - 1982
55	65.163	Vasiliy Kaptyukh, BLR	27.06.1967	1990 - 2004
56	65.153	Dmitriy Shevchenko, RUS	13.05.1968	1990 - 2006
57	65.119	Armin Lemme, GDR	28.10.1955	1979 - 1986
58	65.034	Robert Urbanek, POL	29.04.1987	2011 - 2023
59	65.018	Christoph Harting, GER	04.10.1990	2013 - 2023
60	65.004	Matthew Denny, AUS	02.06.1996	2016 - 2023
61	64.984	Dmytro Kovtsun, UKR	29.09.1955	1979 - 1993
62	64.971	Attila Horváth, HUN	28.07.1967	1988 - 1999
63	64.964	Wolfgang Warnemünde, GDR	08.05.1953	1977 - 1984
64	64.955	Alex Rose, SAM	17.11.1991	2016 - 2023
65	64.950	Georgiy Kolnootchenko, BLR	07.05.1959	1980 - 1990
66	64.923	Uladzimir Dubrovchik, BLR	07.01.1972	1993 - 2001
67	64.883	Benn Harradine, AUS	14.10.1982	2005 - 2017
68	64.837	Rutger Smith, NED	09.07.1981	2002 - 2016
69	64.782	Roland Varga, HUN / CRO	22.10.1977	2000 - 2011
70	64.763	Lois Maikel Martínez, CUB / ESP	03.06.1981	2002 - 2020
71	64.718	Alfred "Al" Oerter, USA	19.09.1936	1966 - 1985
72	64.716	Volodymyr Zinchenko, UKR	25.07.1959	1980 - 1996
73	64.695	Daniel Jasinski, GER	05.08.1989	2012 - 2023
74	64.648	Pentti Kahma, FIN	03.12.1943	1971 - 1976
75	64.615	Adam Setliff, USA	15.12.1969	1993 - 2003
76	64.589	Sam Mattis, USA	19.03.1994	2016 - 2023
77	64.481	Svein Inge Valvik, NOR	20.09.1956	1979 - 1996
78	64.473	Gábor Máté, HUN	09.02.1979	2000 - 2008
79	64.419	Jorge Yadian Fernández, CUB	02.10.1987	2008 - 2023
80	64.344	John van Reenen, RSA	26.03.1947	1969 - 1986
81	64.344	Ihor Duginyets, UKR	20.05.1956	1977 - 1989
82	64.316	Alin Alexandru Firfirica, ROU	03.11.1995	2016 - 2023
83	64.244	Vikas Gowda, IND	05.07.1983	2004 - 2015
84	64.228	Velko Velev, BUL	04.01.1948	1974 - 1985
85	64.226	Hilmar Hoßfeld, GDR	18.01.1954	1980 - 1985
86	64.213	Iosif Nagy, ROU	20.11.1946	1973 - 1985

Table 18 (continued from previous page)

	Men's Best Discus Throwers Using TOP-50 Throw Avg			
	as of 18.09.2023			
Pos	Dist (m)	Athlete	DOB	Active
87	64.176	Märt Israel, EST	23.09.1983	2005 - 2014
88	64.167	Andy Bloom, USA	11.08.1973	1995 - 2004
89	64.166	Bogdan Pishchalnikov, RUS	26.08.1982	2005 - 2012
90	64.128	Niklas Arrhenius, SWE / USA	10.09.1982	2004 - 2022
91	64.101	Casey Malone, USA	06.04.1977	2000 - 2013
92	64.086	Marco Martino, ITA	21.02.1960	1982 - 1991
93	64.023	Mauricio Ortega, COL	04.08.1994	2014 - 2023
94	63.916	Martin Kupper, EST	31.05.1989	2013 - 2020
95	63.886	Mason Finley, USA	07.10.1990	2012 - 2021
96	63.852	Julian Wruck, AUS	06.07.1991	2011 - 2015
97	63.734	Bradley Cooper, BAH	30.06.1957	1979 - 1988
98	63.719	Libor Malina, CZE	14.06.1973	1996 - 2010
99	63.698	Timo Tompuri, FIN	09.06.1969	1998 - 2005
100	63.692	Vésteinn Hafsteinsson, ISL	12.12.1960	1983 - 2000
101	63.661	Victor Hogan, RSA	25.07.1989	2011 - 2023
102	63.653	Apostolos Parellis, CYP	24.07.1985	2012 - 2022
103	63.643	Sergey Lyakhov, RUS	01.03.1968	1988 - 2001
104	63.595	Andreas Seelig, GER	06.07.1970	1995 - 2001
105	63.569	Adewale Olukoju, NGR	27.07.1968	1988 - 1996
106	63.546	Alois Hannecker, FRG	10.07.1961	1983 - 1990
107	63.530	Ion Zamfirache, ROU	23.08.1953	1976 - 1987
108	63.475	David Wrobel, GER	13.02.1991	2014 - 2023
109	63.413	Ola Stunes Isene, NOR	29.01.1995	2018 - 2022
110	63.410	Markus Münch, GER	13.06.1986	2009 - 2017
111	63.401	Guðni Valur Guðnason, ISL	11.10.1995	2015 - 2023
112	63.377	Aleksey Khudyakov, RUS	31.03.1995	2016 - 2023
113	63.372	Dariusz Juzyszyn, POL	29.03.1957	1978 - 1988
114	63.357	Ferenc Tégla, HUN	15.07.1947	1969 - 1984
115	63.352	Andrew Evans, USA	25.01.1991	2013 - 2023
116	63.309	Werner Hartmann, FRG	20.04.1959	1978 - 1988
117	63.301	Costel Grasu, ROU	05.07.1967	1991 - 1999
118	63.262	Kamen Dimitrov, BUL	18.01.1962	1983 - 1991
119	63.242	Reggie Jagers, USA	13.08.1994	2015 - 2022
120	63.235	Hein-Direck Neu, FRG	13.02.1944	1970 - 1980
121	63.229	Chad Wright, JAM	25.03.1991	2012 - 2023
122	63.227	Carl Brown, USA	11.02.1970	1999 - 2005
123	63.214	Nick Sweeney, IRL	26.03.1968	1992 - 2004
124	63.196	Géza Fejér, HUN	20.04.1945	1970 - 1979
125	63.191	Omar Ahmed El Ghazaly, EGY	09.02.1984	2004 - 2012
126	63.169	Viktor Butenko, RUS	10.03.1993	2013 - 2019
127	63.101	Jason Young, USA	27.05.1981	2002 - 2012
128	63.100	Georgiy Taushanski, BUL	26.12.1957	1982 - 1990
129	63.090	Siegfried Pachale, GDR	24.10.1949	1972 - 1976
130	63.059	Aleksandr Borichevski, RUS	25.06.1970	1994 - 2008

Table 19

Pos	Dist (M)	Athlete	DOB	Active
	Men's Best Discus Throwers Using TOP-100 Throw Avg			
	as of 18.09.2023			
1	69.277	Virgilijus Alekna, LTU	13.02.1972	1998 - 2012
2	68.721	Daniel Ståhl, SWE	27.08.1992	2016 - 2023
3	68.684	Gerd Kanter, EST	06.05.1979	2004 - 2013
4	67.936	Lars Riedel, GER	28.06.1967	1991 - 2006
5	67.877	Mac Wilkins, USA	15.11.1950	1975 - 1989
6	67.485	Luis Mariano Delís, CUB	06.12.1957	1979 - 1989
7	67.456	Robert Harting, GER	18.10.1984	2005 - 2017
8	67.381	Imrich Bugár, CZE	14.04.1955	1978 - 1988
9	67.277	Wolfgang Schmidt, GDR / FRG / GER	16.01.1954	1975 - 1992
10	67.053	Piotr Małachowski, POL	07.06.1983	2006 - 2019
11	66.898	Andrius Gudžius, LTU	14.02.1991	2014 - 2023
12	66.698	Jürgen Schult, GDR / GER	11.05.1960	1980 - 2000
13	66.591	Rickard Bruch, SWE	02.07.1946	1969 - 1984
14	66.537	Fedrick Dacres, JAM	28.02.1994	2014 - 2023
15	66.463	John Powell, USA	25.06.1947	1973 - 1987
16	66.431	Art Burns, USA	19.07.1954	1979 - 1987
17	66.132	Knut Hjeltnes, NOR	08.12.1951	1977 - 1989
18	66.077	Kristjan Čeh, SLO	17.02.1999	2018 - 2023
19	66.057	Róbert Fazekas, HUN	18.08.1975	1998 - 2012
20	66.041	Zoltán Kővágó, HUN	10.04.1979	2000 - 2018
21	65.926	Lukas Weißhaidinger, AUT	20.02.1992	2015 - 2023
22	65.730	Mario Pestano, ESP	08.04.1978	2001 - 2014
23	65.724	Frantz Kruger, RSA / FIN	22.05.1975	1998 - 2009
24	65.626	Aleksander Tammert, EST	02.02.1973	1996 - 2012
25	65.586	Romas Ubartas, LTU	26.05.1960	1981 - 2001
26	65.490	Ehsan Hadadi, IRI	21.01.1985	2005 - 2019
27	65.407	Juan Martínez Brito, CUB	17.05.1958	1979 - 1992
28	65.406	Géjza Valent, CZE	03.10.1953	1981 - 1989
29	65.139	Yennifer Frank Casañas, CUB / ESP	18.10.1978	1999 - 2016
30	65.134	Rolf Danneberg, FRG	01.03.1953	1982 - 1990
31	65.129	Michael Möllenbeck, GER	12.12.1969	1993 - 2008
32	64.997	Simon Pettersson, SWE	03.01.1994	2017 - 2023
33	64.917	Martin Wierig, GER	10.06.1987	2009 - 2022
34	64.738	Mike Buncic, USA	25.07.1962	1984 - 1996
35	64.682	Alwin Wagner, FRG	11.08.1950	1977 - 1990
36	64.650	Vaclovas Kidykas, LTU	17.10.1961	1985 - 1999
37	64.588	Markku Tuokko, FIN	24.06.1951	1973 - 1983
38	64.587	Jarred Rome, USA	21.12.1976	2000 - 2013
39	64.520	Ludvík Daněk, CZE	06.01.1937	1964 - 1978
40	64.511	Jason Tunks, CAN	07.05.1975	1996 - 2009

Table 19 (continued from previous page)

Men's Best Discus Throwers Using TOP-100 Throw Avg
as of 18.09.2023

Pos	Dist (M)	Athlete	DOB	Active
41	64.478	Robert Urbanek, POL	29.04.1987	2011 - 2023
42	64.426	Anthony Washington, USA	16.01.1966	1988 - 2000
43	64.412	Philip Milanov, BEL	06.07.1991	2014 - 2023
44	64.385	Erik Cadée, NED	15.02.1984	2009 - 2018
45	64.354	Yuriy Dumchev, RUS	05.08.1958	1979 - 1992
46	64.321	Ian Waltz, USA	15.04.1977	1998 - 2011
47	64.204	Art Swarts, USA	14.02.1945	1972 - 1992
48	64.087	Attila Horváth, HUN	28.07.1967	1987 - 1999
49	64.055	Jay Silvester, USA	27.08.1937	1963 - 1976
50	64.040	Stefan Fernholm, SWE	02.07.1959	1983 - 1996
51	63.997	John Godina, USA	31.05.1972	1992 - 2008
52	63.878	Dmytro Kovtsun, UKR	29.09.1955	1978 - 1995
53	63.795	Erik de Bruin, NED	25.05.1963	1984 - 1993
54	63.770	Roland Varga, HUN / CRO	22.10.1977	1999 - 2016
55	63.764	Benn Harradine, AUS	14.10.1982	2005 - 2018
56	63.722	Traves Smikle, JAM	07.05.1992	2012 - 2023
57	63.721	Vasiliy Kaptyukh, BLR	27.06.1967	1988 - 2005
58	63.688	Ben Plucknett, USA	13.04.1954	1976 - 1989
59	63.654	Kenneth Stadel, USA	19.02.1952	1973 - 1988
60	63.609	Wolfgang Warnemünde, GDR	08.05.1953	1976 - 1986
61	63.518	Alfred "Al" Oerter, USA	19.09.1936	1962 - 1986
62	63.471	Gábor Máté, HUN	09.02.1979	1999 - 2008
63	63.464	Jorge Yadian Fernández, CUB	02.10.1987	2008 - 2023
64	63.463	Christoph Harting, GER	04.10.1990	2010 - 2023
65	63.462	Daniel Jasinski, GER	05.08.1989	2011 - 2023
66	63.461	Lawrence Okoye, GBR	06.10.1991	2011 - 2023
67	63.429	Pentti Kahma, FIN	03.12.1943	1969 - 1977
68	63.382	Rutger Smith, NED	09.07.1981	2002 - 2016
69	63.371	Lois Maikel Martínez, CUB / ESP	03.06.1981	2002 - 2022
70	63.367	Dmitriy Shevchenko, RUS	13.05.1968	1987 - 2007
71	63.337	Niklas Arrhenius, SWE / USA	10.09.1982	2004 - 2022
72	63.318	Svein Inge Valvik, NOR	20.09.1956	1978 - 1999
73	63.304	Matthew Denny, AUS	02.06.1996	2014 - 2023
74	63.278	Märt Israel, EST	23.09.1983	2004 - 2015
75	63.244	Velko Velev, BUL	04.01.1948	1973 - 1986
76	63.201	Sam Mattis, USA	19.03.1994	2014 - 2023

Table 20

Men's Best Discus Throwers Using Top-10 Throws Avg One Season
as of 31.10.2023

1	70.904	Virgilijus Alekna, LTU			2000
1	73.88	Kaunas LTU	1	NC (77)	8/3/2000
2	72.35	Kaunas LTU		NC (77)	8/3/2000
3	71.12	Zürich SUI	1	Weltklasse	8/11/2000
4	70.60	Zürich SUI		Weltklasse	8/11/2000
5	70.42	Zürich SUI		Weltklasse	8/11/2000
6	70.39	Tartu EST	1	Sule (36)	6/11/2000
7	70.26	Zürich SUI		Weltklasse	8/11/2000
8	70.22	Kaunas LTU		NC (77)	8/3/2000
9	70.06	Tartu EST		Sule (36)	6/11/2000
10	69.74	Chemnitz GER	1	Erdgas	7/22/2000
2	**70.728**	**Kristjan Čeh, SLO**			**2023**
1	71.86	Jõhvi EST	1	Heino Lipp (15)	6/16/2023
2	71.70	Jõhvi EST		Heino Lipp (15)	6/16/2023
3	71.19	Jõhvi EST		Heino Lipp (15)	6/16/2023
4	70.89	Doha QAT	1	Diamond/DL	5/5/2023
5	70.70	Doha QAT		Diamond/DL	5/5/2023
6	70.54	Velenje SLO	1	NC	7/9/2023
7	70.32	ar-Rabāṭ MAR	1	MohammedVI/DL	5/28/2023
8	70.07	ar-Rabāṭ MAR		MohammedVI/DL	5/28/2023
9	70.02	Budapest HUN	2	WCh (19)	8/21/2023
10	69.99	Jõhvi EST	1	Jõhvi Discus	8/10/2023
3	**70.586**	**Gerd Kanter, EST**			**2007**
1	72.02	Salinas, California USA	1c1	comp 1	5/3/2007
2	70.93	Helsingborg SWE	1		6/28/2007
3	70.92	Kaunas LTU	2	Kaunas 2007	7/25/2007
4	70.73	Helsingborg SWE			6/28/2007
5	70.52	Salinas, California USA		comp 1	5/3/2007
6	70.36	Kópavogur ISL	1		7/8/2007
7	70.16	Helsingborg SWE	1		8/11/2007
8	70.14	Helsingborg SWE			6/28/2007
9	70.12	Valga EST	1	BIGBANK	6/5/2007
10	69.96	Kópavogur ISL			7/8/2007
4	**70.546**	**Daniel Ståhl, SWE**			**2019**
1	71.86	Bottnaryd SWE	1	Bottnarydskastet	6/29/2019
2	70.89	Varberg SWE	1	Varberg / Folksam GP	7/15/2019
3	70.78	Varberg SWE		Varberg / Folksam GP	7/15/2019
4	70.56	Doha QAT	1	Diamond/DL	5/3/2019
5	70.49	Doha QAT		Diamond/DL	5/3/2019
6	70.37	Varberg SWE		Varberg / Folksam GP	7/15/2019
7	70.36	Varberg SWE		Varberg / Folksam GP	7/15/2019
8	70.32	Doha QAT		Diamond/DL	5/3/2019
9	69.94	ar-Rabāṭ MAR	2	Mohammed VI/DL	6/16/2019
10	69.89	Helsingborg SWE	1	Club Ch	6/26/2019

Table 20 (continued from previous page)

Men's Best Discus Throwers Using Top-10 Throws Avg One Season
as of 31.10.2023

5	70.453	Kristjan Čeh, SLO			2022
1	71.27	Birmingham GBR	1	British GP/DL	5/21/2022
2	71.23	Székesfehérvár HUN	1	Gyulai (12)	8/8/2022
3	71.13	Eugene, Oregon USA	1	WCh (18)	7/19/2022
4	70.72	Roma ITA	1	Golden Gala (42)/DL	6/9/2022
5	70.51	Eugene, Oregon USA		WCh (18)	7/19/2022
6	70.35	Székesfehérvár HUN		Gyulai (12)	8/8/2022
7	70.02	Stockholm SWE	1	Bauhaus (56)/DL	6/30/2022
8	69.91	Velenje SLO	1	NC	6/25/2022
9	69.71	Roma ITA		Golden Gala (42)/DL	6/9/2022
10	69.68	ar-Rabāṭ MAR	1	Mohammed VI/DL	6/5/2022
6	70.149	Daniel Ståhl, SWE			2023
1	71.46	Budapest HUN	1	WCh (19)	8/21/2023
2	71.45	Jõhvi EST	2	Heino Lipp (15)	6/16/2023
3	70.93	Sollentuna SWE	1	Sollentuna / Folksam GP	6/11/2023
4	70.38	Turku FIN	1	PNG (61)	6/13/2023
5	70.25	Karlstad SWE	1	Karlstad / Folksam GP	7/5/2023
6	69.80	Sollentuna SWE	1	LAG-SM	7/8/2023
7	69.63	Turku FIN		PNG (61)	6/13/2023
8	69.37	Budapest HUN		WCh (19)	8/21/2023
9	69.21	ar-Rabāṭ MAR	2	MohammedVI/DL	5/28/2023
10	69.01	Norrköping SWE	1	Tjalves Diskusgala	5/18/2023
7	70.130	Gerd Kanter, EST			2006
1	73.38	Helsingborg SWE	1		9/4/2006
2	72.30	Helsingborg SWE			9/4/2006
3	70.51	Helsingborg SWE			9/4/2006
4	70.43	Helsingborg SWE			9/4/2006
5	69.59	Tallinn EST	1	BIGBANK	8/30/2006
6	69.58	Tallinn EST	1	NC (89)	7/21/2006
7	69.46	Helsingborg SWE			9/4/2006
8	69.05	Tartu EST	1	BIGBANK	8/1/2006
9	68.53	Tallinn EST		BIGBANK	8/30/2006
10	68.47	Stuttgart GER	2	WAF	9/9/2006
8	70.130	Gerd Kanter, EST			2009
1	71.64	Kohila EST	1	BIGBANK	6/25/2009
2	70.92	Kohila EST		BIGBANK	6/25/2009
3	70.84	Chula Vista, California USA	1	WRC	4/28/2009
4	69.99	Helsingborg SWE	1	IFK	9/6/2009
5	69.93	Kohila EST		BIGBANK	6/25/2009
6	69.86	Chula Vista, California USA	1	WRC	5/5/2009
7	69.70	Los Realejos, Tenerife ESP	1cA	EP-w (9)	3/15/2009
8	69.51	Växjö SWE	1 (i)		3/22/2009
9	69.47	La Jolla, California USA	1	WRC	5/12/2009
10	69.44	Helsingborg SWE		IFK	9/6/2009

Table 20 (continued from previous page)

Men's Best Discus Throwers Using Top-10 Throws Avg One Season

as of 31.10.2023

9	70.072	Virgilijus Alekna, LTU			2005
1	70.67	Madrid ESP	1	Meeting Madrid (23)	7/16/2005
2	70.61	Tallinn EST	1	Tammert	9/16/2005
3	70.58	Réthymno GRE	1	Vardinoyiánnia (21)	7/10/2005
4	70.53	Lausanne SUI	1	Athletissima	7/5/2005
5	70.17	Helsinki FIN	1	WCh (10)	8/7/2005
6	69.97	Madrid ESP		Meeting Madrid (23)	7/16/2005
7	69.86	Réthymno GRE		Vardinoyiánnia (21)	7/10/2005
8	69.57	Hengelo NED	1	FBK-Games (23)	5/29/2005
9	69.54	Hengelo NED		FBK-Games (23)	5/29/2005
10	69.22	Sheffield GBR	1	British GP	8/21/2005
10	**70.064**	**Gerd Kanter, EST**			**2008**
1	71.88	Salinas, California USA	1cA	comp A	5/8/2008
2	70.38	Chula Vista, California USA	1	CV Throws	5/2/2008
3	70.32	Helsingborg SWE	1	WRC	9/6/2008
4	70.23	Helsingborg SWE		WRC	9/6/2008
5	69.95	Helsingborg SWE	1	Kasttävling	7/30/2008
6	69.91	Tallinn EST	1	BIGBANK	8/31/2008
7	69.62	Turnov CZE	2	Daněk Memorial (10)	5/20/2008
8	69.54	Chula Vista, California USA		CV Throws	5/2/2008
9	69.53	Valga EST	1	BIGBANK	6/15/2008
10	69.28	Valga EST		BIGBANK	6/15/2008

Table 21

Pos	Avg	Name	DOB	Period
		Season 2021 Top 10 Throws Average		
1	69.401	Daniel Ståhl, SWE	8/27/1992	2021
2	67.885	Kristjan Čeh,SLO	2/17/1999	2021
3	67.111	Andrius Gudžius, LTU	2/14/1991	2021
4	66.537	Lukas Weißhaidinger, AUT	2/20/1992	2021
5	66.461	Simon Pettersson, SWE	1/3/1994	2021
6	65.709	Alex Rose, SAM	11/17/1991	2021
7	65.555	Lawrence Okoye, GBR	10/6/1991	2021
8	65.196	Fedrick Dacres, JAM	2/28/1994	2021
9	64.888	Daniel Jasinski, GER	8/5/1989	2021
10	64.271	Reggie Jagers, USA	8/13/1994	2021
11	64.257	Mauricio Ortega, COL	8/4/1994	2021
12	63.996	Kord Ferguson, USA	6/19/1995	2021
13	63.987	Christoph Harting, GER	10/4/1990	2021
14	63.828	David Wrobel, GER	2/13/1991	2021
15	63.763	János Huszák, HUN	2/5/1992	2021
16	63.427	Brian Williams, USA	12/18/1994	2021
17	63.343	Róbert Szikszai, HUN	9/30/1994	2021
18	63.317	Philip Milanov, BEL	7/6/1991	2021

www.ingramcontent.com/pod-product-compliance
Lightning Source LLC
Chambersburg PA
CBHW051311020426
42333CB00027B/3297